# WISE UP

## POWER, WISDOM, AND THE OLDER WOMAN

BARBARA SCULLY

*For Nor.*

# CONTENTS

# ACKNOWLEDGEMENTS

I always thought writing a book would be a nice, relaxing thing to do. I was wrong. Writing a book is very hard, and I made every mistake possible in the process. But I was helped in no small way by some great friends who were generous with their time, experience, and expertise. And in doing these acknowledgements, I am sure I have left a few people out – please forgive me if I have.

Thank you, Caroline Grace Cassidy, for reading the first draft and putting me wise to the fact that it was only a first draft and to Fiona Looney, who is never less than honest and encouraged me in this endeavour (in a pub in Ahakista – because she definitely won't remember).

Thanks to Cathy Murphy for your forensic attention to detail in that first draft. And to my brother Jim, who also waded through what was a very rough piece of work. Writers Felicity Hayes McCoy and Vanessa O'Loughlin (Sam Blake) thank you for giving me the benefit of your experience and expertise not only on the work but also on how to publish it. And to my published friends Denise

1

Deegan and Eleanor Fitzsimons, who had supported me in this endeavour before it was even conceived.

To my oldest friends, Rita (who features in the book) and Maureen, who have been a part of my life for so long and whose friendship adds such sweetness and depth to my life.

To my friends in media, who have taken me seriously when I am still so unsure of what I am at, trying to write and talk for a living.

To James Wharton – thank you for taking a chance on me and giving me the honour of being the first published author of Zsa Zsa Publishing.

Thank you, Paul (otherwise known as 'Sherwood'), for always believing in me and tolerating most of my plans, except for the very maddest ones. And to my girls… Carla, Roisin and Mia, your constant encouragement and support of my work is just the best, as your collective ability to prevent me from getting ideas above my station.

Finally, to my precious grandchildren, Emie and Max, I hope that someday you might read this in a more equal and peaceful world where the silver-haired crones are visible, valued, and vital.

Barbara Scully

March 2022

# INTRODUCTION

*"Ageing is an extraordinary process where you become the person you should always have been."*

**David Bowie**

Menopause can be a shit show; of that there is no doubt. But after we get through the worst of it, we realise that we have in fact, experienced a huge change of life. And that is what this book is all about. The *change* of life *after* menopause.

If like me, you are a mother, I bet you will have spent many hours telling your teenage or young adult children that they can be anything they choose to be if they work hard enough and put their minds to it. You probably tell them to follow their passions and do things that make their hearts sing. You tell them to be brave and fearless and to go forth and conquer the world. But most of all,

I bet you tell them to be happy. Equally, I bet that this is what you wish most for them: that they are happy and fulfilled wherever their lives may take them.

I have often wondered when women, and not only mothers, stop believing in our own advice when it comes to our own lives. When do we begin to accept less than we should? When is it that we stop seeing our own lives in the same hopeful way as we see those of our kids? When do we stop dreaming of all that there is still to do and all we could still become?

This book is about change, but not just the physical changes that menopause brings. It's also about stripping away the decades of stuff women accumulate as we go through our lives. Once the heavy lifting of parenting is done, once our biology releases its grip on our lives, we are free to look at who we really are. So, in many ways, the change we go through, usually in our fifties, is a kind of reverse metamorphosis. It sometimes feels a bit like the way it felt to get beyond adolescence. Although, unlike our younger selves, we no longer have our whole lives ahead to do with as we wish. But we do have that same dawning awareness that we first experienced when we stood on the threshold of adulthood, the awareness that we are entering a new phase, a time like no other we have experienced before.

During our fifties and early sixties, we will gently lay down many of the labels we have been attached to – mother, daughter, or professional. This presents us with an opportunity to perhaps become someone who, when we examine her carefully, may, in fact, be very closely related to the girl we once were. But now we are embarking on this new phase of life with all our stories, our experiences, our opinions. And it is from these stories and these experiences we gain our wisdom.

Whether you were CEO of a company or a stay-at-home housewife, your experiences, stories, and opinions are important and needed. They are more valuable than a university education. This is a time of life when we need to find our voices to share our experiences and our stories in the public space, whether that's in a mixed social gathering, on social media, or with a wider audience by taking part in the national conversation where women's voices and in particular older women's voices are still largely missing.

It is now that we become aware that time, while not exactly running out, is definitely running down. It is a time to think about what we are going to do in the next decade. Will we have the energy and hopefully the good health to allow us to do these things? And what exactly are these things that we have yet to do? It is now time to bring all that wealth of experience, melt it into the pot of our dreams and create the next phase: potentially the most important phase of your life.

Women's lives meander in a way that men's generally don't. Those of us who become mothers, take far more time out from our jobs and careers to care for our babies than fathers do. Studies show that women still carry the general burden of caring when it comes to elderly parents and others in our families who may need care. So, by the time we reach our fifties, we have probably already managed quite a bit of change in our lives. But much of that change has come about due to our responsibilities to others. Now many of those responsibilities have eased up considerably, particularly in relation to children. The changes you make now, if you're lucky, will be just for you and not driven by someone else's needs.

The freedom that accompanies a completed menopause signals a significant shift in many women's lives. From talking to post-menopausal women, I know that many experience an underlying need to explore parts of themselves that have been parked for decades while they perhaps climbed the career ladder or stayed home and looked after their kids. By the time they reach their late fifties, they may be ready to retire from their career or, if they were housewives, maybe embark on a paid career. They might, for instance, set up a small business, learn a new skill, write a book, make soap, or begin to paint.

Around this age, there is also an increasing realisation that, in order to make the most of the years ahead, good health is going to be vital. For many post-menopausal women, that may involve losing weight and gaining fitness. Of course, we will probably already have discovered that this is not at all as easy as it sounds. Old habits are hard to break. However, as my doctor said to me when I was diagnosed with Type 2 Diabetes at 57,

"You get away with it, until you stop getting away with it." And if we want to make the most of the decades ahead, good health is vital.

Lifestyle change, losing weight and becoming fitter is hard. It took me a diagnosis of diabetes to shift my lardy arse off the sofa and onto the road to retrieving my health. I didn't see that I had a problem until I had a problem. I spent decades making a virtue of hating exercise and being totally comfortable in my own skin. I knew I was fat, but I was body confident. What I didn't see, and avoided confronting, was that I was very unfit. And fitness is key.

Now please don't think for any minute that I have become a marathon runner or someone who dons Lycra and cycles up and down the country. I have not. I am not thin either. But I move every day. I am conscious of what I eat, although that doesn't mean I can't have an occasional treat and often more than occasionally too. But I try now to keep my eye on what I am doing and try not to over-treat myself. I also have to watch my portion sizes continually. However, the benefits of weight loss and fitness have been tremendous and can be summed up in one sentence. I feel younger than I have in about a decade.

I'll explore how I changed my eating habits and overcame my exercise phobia in the "Change of Life" section. It is not a blueprint for change, but it worked for me, and perhaps it will help you find what works for you, should you wish to regain control of your health.

In the chapter "A Woman's Voice", I discuss, among other things, changing your mindset about getting older and working out how to deal with the constant messaging mature women get about fighting ageing. It is the most pointless fight you will ever engage in, although it will relieve you of many hundreds (or perhaps thousands) of euros and take a good sideswipe at your confidence while you're at it.

For many women, confidence is something that seems to decrease over the years, especially if many of those years were spent at home looking after your children. I spent a decade doing just that, and in that time I, like many women, lost a bit of myself. Lost a lot of myself. Well, maybe "lost" is not the right word. Because loss implies permanence, and I think I always knew, if only subliminally, that what I was doing was not forever.

For some women, the opportunity to retire from the world of paid work signals an opportunity to pick up pieces of themselves that they had sacrificed to facilitate work. Either way, it's now time to retrieve those bits of ourselves again. And one of the parts of ourselves that we often lose is confidence, particularly the confidence needed to become something different. I bet I am not the only woman who hears the voice in her head that constantly tells her she's crazy to think she could do that, be that, have that, or go there. Getting that voice to shut up is not easy, but you can learn to literally tell it to do so. To shut up.

Staying at home, caring for children and running the domestic life of a family gets no recognition in society, so it's hardly surprising that the years spent being a housewife rob women of confidence. Moreover, if you have been in a corporate workplace, you may have lost touch with who you really are, as you have spent decades being whatever it is you do for a living. In fact, if there was one free gift I could have packaged with this book, it would be the gift of self-confidence.

Remember when you were young and dreamed of your life and how it would pan out? Maybe your vision was of travelling the world, experiencing many different cultures. Maybe it was to climb that corporate ladder, or perhaps it was to have a partner and children, or a combination of all of those and more. But regardless of what your dream was, I am sure you had a vision of how you wanted your life to pan out.

However, as we go through life, most of us discover that it doesn't always pan out exactly how we envisioned it. Even if you eventually got to the position you had been dreaming of, it's more likely than not that you took a route that was somewhat different to the one you imagined you would take. But you survived. You amended your vision, trimmed your sails, and you got on with it.

And now a lot of it is done or almost done. Your kids may have left home, your mortgage will eventually be paid off, and you will retire from your career. (Although if, like us, you took out a mortgage when you were forty, you wouldn't want to wait until that's paid off, as you are likely to be a bit less energetic by then. Buy when you are young, people, buy when you are young.) And if the fates are with you, you will still have energy and good health to explore other options. Menopause means change, and change means opportunity.

Now is the time to review the decades you have lived, to laugh at the absurdities, to recognise the tough times and to congratulate yourself for making it this far. Because, regardless of what our society might say (or more often not say), your experiences are important and not just to you. Women have long recognised the power of sharing our stories, albeit in safe female spaces. We learn from each other. We draw strength from each other.

As we cruise towards our sixties and even our seventies, we need to clarify how we want this phase of life, this freedom to be. These really are golden years, but the clock is ticking, and we need to make sure we don't waste them. So, start dreaming. Now. Dream of where you want to go (yeah, I know it's a cliché, but I do mean the bucket list stuff), dream of where you want to live and, more importantly, HOW you want to live. And dream of the things you want to do and to achieve. As you learn to let your mind stretch to accommodate dreams, no matter how far-fetched and impossible, you might find that these midlife dreams are actually not so different from the dreams you had as a kid. And that right there is the beauty of this.

As I said, when you begin to explore other options, you may have the feeling that you are connecting right back to the girl you were once were. This can be such a joyous reunion, but be warned it will be tainted; tainted with regrets for things you think you did wrong, for opportunities not taken, for losses you have experienced. Nevertheless, all of those things will now make you wiser than you have ever been before. They should drive you forward without fear of failure or judgement. That's not to say you won't fail or be judged, but you will probably already have experienced these and a myriad of other negative experiences, and you have survived. So, unlike when you were a child or a teenager, failure and ridicule hold no fear for you. And that is another precious freedom right there.

Menopause is a transit lounge, not a destination. It means that you are on your way to somewhere different but stuck on a bit of a layover. Menopause is a portal. Sometimes a long, tortuous one but a gateway to what could be the most satisfying time of your life. It's up to you to choose where the journey will take you. However, make no mistake; you are travelling, girl. You are moving on. Make the most of it. Sing your song loud and clear. Take opportunities. Take risks. Remember all the stuff you told your kids as they embarked on adulthood and start following your own advice. I am not only suggesting big changes; small ones are just as important, as long they are what you want to do.

I hope that this book will shine a light for you on your own life so that you can see just how powerful you can be. While I don't have a 12-step method you can follow, I hope that if I share some of my experiences, you will begin to believe that any change is possible.

But much as I want this book to inspire and motivate you, what I want most is for you to enjoy it. I hope you will laugh at least a few times while reading. Because when all is said and done, life is something not to be taken too seriously. Even when it is serious.

# SO, WHO ARE YOU?

Before we prepare for what may just be the most important phase of our lives, it's important to have a look back over the decades that have gone before. A kind of stocktake of where we have been and what we have done. Because *real* wisdom will only come from understanding our stories and experiences, owning them – the good and the bad – and knowing that all that we have experienced up to now has played a huge part in who we are.

*Our stories are like the squares on a patchwork quilt that we gather around ourselves as we go forward, keeping us warm, reminding us that we have loved and are loved, and, most importantly, that we have lived. Everything we have experienced prepares us for what is to come, regardless of how our lives have played out and although perhaps we may not always have thrived, we have survived. We are still here.*

*In the following chapters, I will share some of the stories and defining elements of each of the decades I have lived thus far. Because they have all played a part in bringing me to this place, they are all part of my story.*

*Your stories are different. But this kind of approach might be very useful for you when you undertake a similar stocktake of your life thus far.*

# THE GOLDEN TWENTIES

*"We all go a little mad, sometimes."*

**Norman Bates,** *Psycho*

## TURNING TWENTY... SORT OF.

I don't remember turning twenty. Nothing. Not one memory at all. So, I am guessing it wasn't a momentous occasion. January 1982. Ireland was a dull place in the teeth of a recession and that January, it was also in the grip of a blizzard, which arrived a few days before my birthday. The country was frozen to a near standstill, with power cuts adding to the isolation of villages and towns already cut off from the rest of the world, wrapped in a thick blanket of white silence. It was bleak – on all fronts.

However, I had a job working for JWT, Ireland's largest tour operator at the time. During this blizzard,

I remember struggling to get into work. There were no trains, my normal mode of transport into the city, and no buses either. Undeterred, I stood on the main road and hitched a lift. Yep, I happily jumped into a car with a stranger who was going to try to negotiate slippery roads that were too dangerous for public transport, all just in case someone needed to book a holiday. I remember being surprised to find there was only me and one other eejit who made it to the office that day.

In hindsight, it was just as well I had no party planned; no one could have made it through the snow that was crippling the country. However, unlike all your other "roundy" birthdays, your twentieth isn't a significant milestone as it is completely overshadowed by one's twenty-first… or even one's eighteenth.

You won't be surprised to hear that I had turned 18, two years previously, in January 1980. I had just started my new job, but my heart and my social life were immersed in my local area, of Dun Laoghaire, a seaside town on the south side of Dublin city that was said at the time to have the highest proportion of young people of any town in Ireland. It was a great place to "come of age".

I desperately wanted an eighteenth birthday party but, having just started working and earning the princely sum of £43 per week, there was no way I could afford even the most modest of bashes. And back in those days, parents of adult children didn't generally stump up for frivolous incidentals like parties.

However, one night in the local pub, our large group of friends realised that six of us were all going to turn 18 that momentous January. So, we wondered if by clubbing together we could throw a party. We checked out the cost of hiring a room, a bar extension and a DJ and soon realised that even sharing the cost wasn't an option. The dream of a proper party was still beyond our reach. Until that is, someone came up with the brain wave of selling tickets to attend. Yep, we could charge our friends and family to come to our party. And that is just what we did. We had tickets printed, which we sold for £2 each, enabling us to hire a DJ, book a venue and bar extension and, as far as I remember, there was a small amount left in the kitty with which we bought ourselves a birthday round of drinks. It was a massive success, and it set the tone for the years ahead. Life was largely a party to be enjoyed and, if you wanted something badly enough, you could make it happen.

## GREAT EXPECTATIONS

All through my teenage years, I dreamed of being an adult: the freedom, the independence, and the sex. All through the years of struggling with acne, and coming to terms with my changing body and its mysterious functions, as I grappled with studying stuff in which I had little interest and finally, with exams, I dreamed. I dreamed of the time when it would all be over, and I would finally be mistress of my own destiny.

My teens were not that remarkable for someone of my age growing up in Ireland, in that they didn't feature the opposite sex at all. I went to an all-girls secondary school, and, even in junior school, we were kept completely segregated from the boys. So, growing up, I knew no boys other than my brothers. I left school in June 1979, and I had a busy agenda to pursue. And the first item on that agenda was finding a boyfriend.

Turning 18 marked my transition into adulthood far more than my twentieth did. Over the space of one summer, I morphed from schoolgirl to working woman. The world also felt like it was changing, as it usually does with each new decade. The 1980s would be the decade of my twenties, and I couldn't wait. It was the era of New Romantics, of Duran Duran and Spandau Ballet and the best girl group ever, Bananarama.

The so-called second wave of feminism had arrived in Ireland in the 1970s and given women and girls, even those of us who were closeted with the nuns in a convent school, the idea that we could have it all. This brave new world of women's liberation meant that we could look forward to a great career, owning a car and an apartment and, in due course, also getting married and having children. But the marriage and children bit was pretty far down the road as far as I was concerned. This was the era of "power dressing", shoulder pads and big hair. Women looked powerful, although they were still largely confined to support roles in the workforce and, even where they competed equally with men, they were still (legally) paid less.

When I left school, the career options for girls were mainly secretarial. In fact, it's a bit of a paradox that the only women I was aware of running businesses were the nuns who ran schools and hospitals. They did their own version of power dressing, swooshing up and down the school corridors in their voluminous black habits and veils. Way more intimidating than shoulder pads and big hair but devoid of any glamour, which was an essential element of power dressing.

The summer I left school, I remember thinking I might like to travel for a year before settling down to earn my living, but my dear mother put paid to that idea, thinking it might unsettle me and I might never return to "normal" life. She may have had a point and, although I enrolled in the requisite secretarial course, I never dreamed of being someone's secretary. I dreamed of working in the travel business. So, just before my eighteenth birthday, I began my first real job, selling holidays for tour operator JWT.

My eighteenth birthday not only marked the beginning of my nineteenth year on the planet, but it was the threshold over which I passed into the decade of my twenties, albeit two years early. I couldn't wait to get started on my life.

And that is key to understanding your twenties. As you embark on this formative decade, you are unwavering in your belief that you will be the author of your own story. The world was my oyster to do with as I wanted. As I headed towards twenty, I was finally in control. I had the job I had craved, I had my own money – not a lot of it, but it was mine, all mine to do with as I pleased – and yes, of course, I paid up at home, but otherwise it was all mine.

Most of all, I finally had a boyfriend with whom I was in love. Now, OK, I know I was a bit late to the boyfriend party… I blame that on the nuns. But we all remember our first love, and if you are lucky (like I was), it is a positive, special experience. You will always remember the first time you had that fizzy feeling of excitement at just the sight of someone you thought was the most gorgeous creature you had ever laid eyes on. The passion and the excitement of it all was just delicious.

So, your twenties is the decade that often begins with the greatest of expectations. You are invincible and, unless you have had to deal with some trauma in your young life, you are full of positivity and are sure that life will pan out exactly as you want it to. It's a heady time. All the firsts are there – first job, first love, first holiday (without your parents), and first car. Your dreams are all vivid and bright. In addition, in the 1980s, we had the fabulous soundtrack to match.

Before I recount some of the defining episodes of my twenties, I have to begin with one of the most defining things about my life then and now, my height.

# THE STORIES

## *You're Tall*

I met someone once who knew me from the telly (which I do a small bit of), and she greeted me with, "you're just like you are on the telly, only much taller." I am six feet tall, which is not that remarkable today but believe me, forty years ago, when I reached my zenith, it was quite something.

I think it was when I was in primary school that I first realised that I was taller than the average girl or boy. And it was when I began my life long search for clothes long enough, something that has only recently been resolved with the introduction of "tall ranges" in women's clothes.

When I was a young girl, like all girls in the '60s and '70s, I had to wear woolly tights to school in the winter. I never ever owned a pair that fitted me. I pulled them on and up, and things seemed fine until I began to walk. The more steps I took, the further south my tights migrated. So I developed a winter walking style all my own – which involved two normal strides and one giant one as I attempted to subtly manoeuvre the crotch back to where it belonged. It was a losing battle. By the time I arrived at school, my tights had travelled south towards my knees, where thankfully they got stuck, saving me any obvious embarrassment other than the wrinkled gathering of spare tight at each ankle!

This childhood trauma meant that I have never worn tights as an adult woman. The weather could be minus two degrees outside, and I will be in trousers or leggings. Otherwise, if the occasion absolutely demands a dress, I may even be bare-legged.

Of course, by the time I moved into secondary school, my height meant that I was the hanger of pictures, the closer of windows and even the pusher of the huge equipment that was needed back then to play audio and videotapes. The nuns equated height with strength for some reason. I also got to hold all the sex education charts of male and female anatomy during our technicolour sex education classes – brought to us by a nun. In our religion class. No wonder my generation can be a bit odd in the head when it comes to sex.

## "The Big One"

My PE teacher tried to press-gang me into all kinds of sports in which my height might be an advantage, including long jump, javelin and shot put (oh yes, that old height and strength thing again). I was useless at all of them. I finally found a place on the basketball team but, as I couldn't run to catch a bus, my job was never to go too far into defence so that I could make it back to the basket when the game turned around. My job was to merely score baskets. I was only a passable basket scorer most days, but occasionally I had a really good game.

One game when I was 15 years old stands out in

my memory; I wasn't quite on fire, but I was definitely smouldering and causing problems for the opposition. We were playing away at another girls' school on the other side of the city, and they had a cool young American guy as their coach. He stood on the sidelines and got more and more frustrated as our score kept climbing, thanks mainly to yours truly.

"Mark the big one, mark the big one," he kept shouting.

Initially, I suppressed my irritation as I enjoyed the rare experience of actually doing what I was meant to do on the court. But he said it one time too many, so I called time out.

I went over to him, standing as straight as I could and said, "I have a number on my skirt (oh yes, no shorts for nice convent-educated girls playing sports back in the 70s), and it is also on the back of my shirt. If you want to refer to me, please use my number. I am not 'the big one.'"

I remember how stunned he was. But it worked. He changed his tune and used my number for the rest of the match.

I think that, although I didn't realise it until much later, that may have been the first time I ever experienced the power that comes with height. It shouldn't, but it does.

Having said that, it didn't mean that I wasn't christened with various names when I was younger. I remember walking home from school one day, and a group of boys shouted, "Jaysus, you are like the Towering Inferno"; I wasn't sure if it was a compliment or not. On reflection, as it came from a movie about a skyscraper on fire, I thought probably not. When I began working in the travel business, I was known as Big Bird or BB for short by some of my colleagues.

However, it wasn't only the nuns who got confused about what advantages height confers on a body; the general populace did too. I grew up hearing, "oh, you are so tall; you could be a model". Em, no, I couldn't have been a model. I am not built like a model and never have been, except for a short spell after a growth spurt when I was about 14 when I did get very lanky and skinny for a bit. The other thing they say, as the truth dawns that you are a bit roundy, is, "oh, with your height, you can carry a bit of extra weight." Em, no. You are just tall and a bit fat instead of short or average and a bit fat.

Being so tall was the defining factor not only when I went to buy clothes but also when it came to boys. Two things that are extraordinarily important in your twenties. But one of the most important lessons I learned as I raced into adulthood was to NEVER, EVER sit down for the "slow set".

## The Slow Set

Ah, the slow set: a glorious thing now unfortunately consigned to history. The disco lights would slow to a flicker, and the opening bars of 10cc's "I'm Not In Love" would reverberate around the hall (yep, it was usually a sports hall or community centre) and, as the beat slowed down, the girls would all take to the seating around the walls. The lads would make their way nervously through a fug of cigarette smoke to their chosen one to ask her to dance.

I could never take a seat with the rest of the girls because, as soon as I did, one of the smallest fellas in the place would make his way over to me. I could see him steaming towards me like a miniature Titanic cruising towards the iceberg. "Do you want to dance?" he'd mutter as his mates, gathered in a circle, watched on. What to do?

If I said yes and stood up, his mistake would be obvious, and he would be covered in confusion about what to do next. If I politely refused, I risked him getting all shirty and smart for my having the audacity to spurn his advances. So, I never sat down. Which kind of put me with the lads as opposed to the girls. And only very rarely did I get asked to dance.

## First Love

Not getting asked to dance at the local discos was beginning to be a problem, as one of the main aims I had for the summer I left school was finding some boy who was tall enough to accompany me to my Debs.

In Ireland, one's Debs is a very big deal, even back in 1979. Although it takes its name from that very British tradition of a young woman's "debut" into high society, which included being presented to the Monarch, the Irish version is, like so many things in Ireland, a grand excuse for a good party and getting dressed up. It does not involve being presented to anyone, but it does require an escort. Debs balls take place in the autumn after you leave school. So, I had a summer to find a fella, and he had to be over 6' tall.

I first laid eyes on possibly the only tall, handsome guy in Dun Laoghaire early in the summer I left school when I passed him and his friend on the opposite side of the road. He was very tall and had long leather-clad legs, which immediately caught my attention. Once they had passed, I decided to risk a second glance. As I turned around, so did he. Eyes met, and we both laughed. And I fell in love, in the way you do when you are 17. For those last weeks of school, I spend too long daydreaming about Sexy Long Legs. I had found the guy to take me to the Debs. I just had to find out who he was and work out how to meet him.

Once exams were over, we raced out of school for the last time and straight into our futures, which we were sure we would find in Dunelles pub. Located in the basement of the local shopping centre, it was a windowless, dark cavern of a place. It seemed mysterious and exciting. No one who frequented Dunelles was over

30 years of age. It was like a private club for penniless youths. A local musician played almost every night, and his guitar wove the music of Dylan, Young and Croce into my memories of the place. There was magic and lots of cigarette smoke in the air. New York had Studio 54; Dun Laoghaire had Dunelles.

The best spot was a booth with a view of the stairs. From there, the girls and I would play the "whose legs are those" game as they descended into the murky half-light. Sexy Long Legs was a regular and highly popular by all accounts. He seemed to know everyone except me. We smiled at each other and even moved on to a shy 'Hi', but there we got stuck. Summer rolled on, and my main worry was my Debs and the fact that Sexy Long Legs seemed to know every girl in Dun Laoghaire. The clock was ticking. I had to get to know him well enough to get the big ask in before someone else did.

Finally, in late July, I managed to get myself introduced to him by a mutual friend, as my friend Rita and I were waiting for the last bus home. Trying to act cool but feeling very hot under the collar, we boarded the bus; he sat on the seat in front of us and offered me a cigarette. Through a cloud of noxious fumes, I abandoned small talk and got right to the point, conscious that his journey was shorter than mine. (Yes, of course, I had found out where he lived, which was some feat in the days before the internet.)

"Would you fancy coming to my Debs in November," I gushed at him. "Yeah, why not," he answered, "that will be three Debs Balls for me this autumn." It wasn't quite the answer I was looking for. But it was a yes, and I figured he would look great in a tuxedo. I skipped off the bus at my stop and floated all the way home with a mixture of relief and excitement bubbling through my heart.

The next night in Dunelles, I couldn't wait to meet my new friend, my Debs date. In he came and, as he breezed past, the only change was that he now said "Hi Barbara" instead of just "Hi". Slowly, the realisation dawned that my asking him to my Debs had not conferred any new status on our relationship. In fact, I was just last in a queue of three girls with whom he would be doing the same. So, I was trapped in a weird kind of limbo.

Summer faded into autumn, and I continued to try to capture the heart of Sexy Long Legs. My perseverance paid off, and finally, there was the momentous day when he took me on a walk down the pier, where we smoked a joint. Afterwards, we lay on the grass in the park and watched the clouds slowly creep across the blue sky while listening to the twang of bowls from the green nearby. I finally had his full and undivided attention.

And yes, he was indeed a wonderful date at my Debs. He looked very handsome, made me feel less of a giant and brought magic mushrooms to add to the mushroom soup, which added no end of craic to the proceedings.

We dated for over a year, during which we were two of the six conspirators who shared that fabulous eighteenth birthday party.

Our relationship burned bright and sizzled along with great excitement. And I am glad to say that, when it ended, a year or so later, we remained friends. In fact, a couple of decades later, we both ended up living in the same neighbourhood with our respective spouses and children.

He was a good guy who made me feel special, sexy and smart – all the things you want to feel when you are almost twenty. After some years of ill health, he died while I was away in Australia for the birth of my first grandchild. I am still sad that I never got to say goodbye, to attend his funeral or, most of all, to remind him before he died that he was a good guy. A really good guy.

## *Risky Business*

Your late teens and early twenties are the risk-taking years and the years in which you experiment with all kinds of previously forbidden delights. Back in the early 80s, drink was expensive and not generally something your Ma put in her shopping trolley every week, as I have been able to do for decades. My father was a Pioneer. No, that doesn't mean that he explored uncharted territories but that he was a member of… wait for it… The Pioneer Total Abstinence Association of the Sacred Heart. In other words, he was a Catholic who didn't drink and proudly wore a pin on his lapel to proclaim this fact. In reality, my dad hated alcohol and what it did to people. My mother didn't quite share his abhorrence, but suffice to say that in our house, there was probably a bottle of whiskey for when the priest called, sherry for Christmas pudding and brandy to settle a tummy upset.

So, as soon as I started to earn my own money, I began to be able to afford to have a drink on the weekend. Or during the week. Or anytime I liked. I also travelled regularly, so, in my bedroom, I had my own drinks cabinet, which usually contained a bottle of duty-free Bacardi and one of Malibu. The problem with learning about drinking is finding out when enough is enough, and, along the way, we all have mortifying occasions when we make a complete fool of ourselves.

Bacardi once made me puke on the street in San Antonio, Ibiza, which was very uncool (this was before the ladette culture of the 90s); too much Ouzo delivered quite pleasant but unnerving hallucinations in Corfu, and tequila shots made me do all kinds of foolish things right here in Dublin. By your mid-twenties, you should have learned where that sweet point is when you feel very happy and floaty, but before that descends into the chaos of not being able to control your legs or your digestive system.

For women, the sense of invincibility you feel at this age is particularly dangerous. This is because, at the same time, you have possibly yet to learn that the world can be a dangerous place for a woman, especially when you are alone and maybe not quite as alert as usual. When I look back now at some of the things I did, my blood runs cold. I think that perhaps my great height protected me a bit. Most men have a natural physical power over most women because of their greater height and strength. But, at six feet tall, I was probably not worth the risk.

I remember my mother giving out to me for walking home in the early hours, alone through what she considered to be a dodgy part of town. And I remember my answer. "Ma, I am six feet tall with no boobs. If I change my walk I could look like a man. I am fine." My own youngest daughter, who is six foot two, said something similar to me recently.

When I wasn't negotiating mean streets in the early hours but out in a pub or nightclub, my height did cause me to worry somewhat. Because in low light, I thought I could possibly be mistaken for a not particularly good drag queen. As far as I was concerned, six-foot-tall women just didn't exist. I knew no other woman who was even close to my height when I was in my teens and twenties.

## The Sum Of Our Parts

Overall, the advantages of being tall outweighed the disadvantages. I liked the feeling of strength and power it gave me. However, like most young women and indeed girls, I wasted far too much time in my twenties wishing bits of my body were different. If only I had known how fabulous I was. If only we all knew how fabulous we are when we are in our twenties. Instead, like many of you, I would imagine, I wished I were slimmer. I wished that my ankles were thinner, my ears were smaller and less sticky out, my thighs were less ample, and my hair was either curly or straight. Actually, that's a lie. I wished it was curly. I spent hours and hours having my hair permed in the 80s. I so wanted proper curly hair. God gave me the long legs, but she got the width measurement surprisingly wrong. Therefore, in my youth, I felt my legs were at least two sizes too big for the rest of me. God also gifted me with two knees on each leg to compound her error. Of course, I still have big, lumpy knees – only now they match the rest of me.

Another thing I was often told when I was young was, "oh, you are so lucky, being tall, you could wear anything." I heard this so much that I began to believe it. I made some really bad fashion choices in my early twenties. In about 1982, the season's must-have was a satin jumpsuit. Yep, and sure, I could wear anything. Off I went and purchased a purple one in which I thought I was very sophisticated in a *Challenge Anneka* kind of way (Anneka Rice – ask your mother). I decided that a formal Gala Dinner (they were big in corporate Ireland in the '80s) would be the perfect occasion to christen my new outfit: big, permed hair, silver blusher, glitter eye shadow and my purple satin jumpsuit. Off I went, delighted with myself. However, not long into the evening, I began to realise I was having problems standing up straight. If I did, the neck at the back of my suit was pulled downwards with a resultant pulling northwards of the front resulting in a phenomenon that I believe is known as dromedary tarsals. I didn't do much dancing that night.

So, despite the challenges of my great height and big feet, my twenties were motoring along more or less as I had hoped they would. I had fallen in love and out again. I had a job I loved; the pay was awful, but the perks were great. Back in the days when air travel was truly expensive, I could avail myself of free travel to the sunshine resorts of Europe. Now, I know that pales into insignificance when compared to today's young twenty-somethings jaunting all over the world, but in the '80s, I was definitely a jet setter.

Heading towards my mid-twenties, my friends were beginning to get married, and I was merrily content with being single and able to mingle! There were more romances here and there, and my social life was great. All was well in the world. All was going as intended. Then life flung a huge curveball straight at me, hitting me right in the chops.

## Unmarried Mother

On the 28th of July 1987, at the tender age of 25, I became a single mother – or as it was much more delicately referred to back then – An Unmarried Mother; a term which gave the impression that I had somehow managed to achieve the biological miracle of making myself pregnant all by myself.

Three years earlier in Ireland, the schoolgirl Anne Lovett had died alongside her baby in a freezing graveyard in Longford, where she had just given birth. That same year the country was convulsed with the case that became known as The Kerry Babies. Another young single woman, who was known to have been pregnant, was accused of killing not only her own baby but also another baby found on a beach in Kerry, some 80km from her home. It took until 2018 for the wrongly accused woman, Joanne Hayes, to be finally vindicated and receive an apology from the Gardai and the government. This was Ireland in the mid-1980s. It was a cold place for "unmarried mothers" but a place where the fathers (because despite the term, babies can't be made without a man's input) were still completely free of responsibilities should they choose to cut and run. And, more importantly, they were completely free of judgement.

Now I should say that the 28th of July 1987 remains one of the happiest days of my life as I had given birth to the daughter I always knew I would have. Also, I should acknowledge that I had the support of my parents. My brothers were in the picture, too, lending their own unique kind of support.

Anyway, being An Unmarried Mother meant that I suddenly wasn't exactly single with its freedom to pursue the hedonistic lifestyle of those in their mid-twenties, but I clearly wasn't married either. Underpinning this was the fact that I was most definitely outside the respectability circle. I didn't entirely mind this, as I have always been a bit of an anarchist. However, it sure went a long way in making me the "mad feminist" (think I am quoting one of my dear brothers correctly) that I am today.

Although, to be fair, it was more, well, aggressive than that. Being an Unmarried Mother made me hate men. Not because one had made me pregnant and chosen not to involve himself. That suited me fine. No, it was society's views of single parents that made me angry and made me hate men. I didn't know it then, but I had run smack bang into the patriarchy. And the patriarchy thought any woman who became pregnant outside marriage was clearly a slut. You think I'm imagining that, right? After all, it was 1987, I hear you mutter. Well, let me recount just one experience I had, which illustrates exactly what I mean.

After my daughter was born, I was off work on maternity leave, so I was at home. One day I answered the phone; it was for my dad, who was by then retired. It was a pal of his, who, like my dad, was a retired senior public servant. Although this man, my dad's friend, was someone with a degree of public profile. I could only hear my dad's side of the conversation naturally, and it went like this.

"No, that was Barbara".

"No, she isn't working at the moment because, well, erm, she has just had a baby".

"No, no, she didn't get married."

"Oh yes, yes, she does know who the father is".

The tragedy of this story is that I got so angry, but it wasn't for myself because I think I had already internalised the fact that I was now somewhat sullied by lone motherhood. I was angry that my father had been insulted and slighted by this man's judgement.

My father was a conservative man. Telling him that I was pregnant is still something I wish I hadn't had to do because it upset him so much. Although he was a man of few words, I knew he loved me, and I also knew that, despite the fact that I hadn't followed him into the public service, something he really wanted me to do, he was proud of me. After telling him my news, I remember having to listen to him vomiting in the bathroom – that's how deeply upset he was by my' predicament'.

He couldn't speak to me for about three weeks. There was no anger. No recriminations, no lectures. Just a silence that burned through the house as he grappled with this new reality. It was awful. I couldn't afford to move out but was beginning to believe I couldn't stay either.

Then one day, I arrived home early from work. He was in the kitchen making tea. He turned to me and pulled me into a hug, and said, "we will support you; we will stand by you. It'll be OK." The relief was enormous. I knew I couldn't have managed on my own. And he was true to his word. My mother, once she had delivered a half-hearted lecture about my being irresponsible in allowing myself to get pregnant, was quite gung-ho about it all and relished this new adventure.

But society's judgement continued. Looking back now at photos of me from those years, I can see just how incensed I was. I wore my hair really short so that even my large, sticky-out ears were visible. But what was more visible was the expression I wore most of the time, which featured a lot during the punk era in the 70s. It clearly shouted, "Fuck You".

For years, as I struggled to parent my own little person (and no, it wasn't easy even with the great support I had), I was treated to what seemed like an endless stream of debates on the national airwaves about the rise of these "unmarried mothers". Of course, right up into the 1980s and indeed the 1990s, many unmarried mothers were hidden away, down the country or in a Magdalene Laundry or Mother and Baby Home. And now we all know how that panned out for these women and their babies.

Joining the EU (or EEC as it was in 1973) meant that Ireland got a boot up the arse in relation to its treatment of women. A raft of legislation brought, among other things, an end to the marriage bar, which forced women to leave the workforce when they got married.

It also resulted in the introduction of the unmarried mothers' allowance. So, these inconvenient unmarried mothers came out of the shadows and into the light, like an awkward relative at a family wedding. And Ireland worried. These shameless women (like, they had to be shameless, right?) had most likely deliberately gotten pregnant just to claim this allowance and not have to work. Then they would apply for a council house (back in the days when the government actually built social housing). In other words, they would just milk the system and all at the respectable taxpayer's expense.

Then, of course, there was the problem of raising kids without a father – the natural head of any household you understand. These poor kids would no doubt be damaged and turn out to be delinquents, causing endless problems as they became teenagers. Because, obviously, a mother alone cannot successfully raise children.

I listened to this shit for years. Shit that was spouted mainly but not exclusively by politicians, priests, and bishops – all male. It made me mad as hell. I was taking responsibility for my child, teaching her, feeding her, clothing her, and doing the job of two parents. Yet, despite this, somewhere in my subconscious, I began to believe that I was failing. I spent so many years feeling guilty about the damage my reckless behaviour would do to my daughter. That still makes me angry, even all these years later. And I was lucky. I was not from a deprived background, and I had the support of my family, who were great. How women without these two advantages coped and still cope, I don't know.

Being a single parent did have its advantages. We did so much together, just the two of us. And so, we forged a very strong bond. However, I think it may have been hard on her at times. We were very close, and she probably had a ringside seat for much of my emotional turmoil and my man-hating during her early years.

# THE WISDOM TAKEAWAYS

The decade that I had expected to be all about decadence, abandon, wildness, learning, love, sex and growing up was all that. It was huge fun and certainly very exciting. I learned that love is wonderful, as is sex, especially with the right person, which gives it added depth. By the end of the decade, I had learned how to drink with minimal falling down and puking, having first suffered the ignominy of both on numerous occasions.

But I did spend too many hours wishing I looked different. So much time was wasted on wishing for the impossible. Sometimes, we think that almost universal unhappiness with our looks as young women is a new phenomenon. It's not. It may be worse today with Instagram and filters and face tuning, but it has been an aspect of being a young woman for decades.

It was in my teens at that basketball match that I first spoke up for myself when someone, the basketball coach, was being what I considered to be disrespectful. Being tall makes this easier because you can often look the person to whom you are speaking in the eye or, even better, look at them down your nose. In my twenties, I also led a minor revolt in my first job over the non-payment of Christmas bonuses to staff under two years' service even though it was against our contract. It was a small victory, but a victory nonetheless. It's funny, but looking back, I think many of us are much more fearless when we are young. I guess when there is little to lose, you are freer to gamble.

I think bad fashion choices are a necessary rite of passage, too, although the '80s presented us with unique opportunities to not only wear something that didn't really suit us but that also made a big statement as we sparkled and glittered and shoulder-padded about looking very odd. This was the "greed is good" decade when more was more, and good taste got somewhat lost.

In general, my twenties blazed brightly and noisily, but, like fireworks, it burned out somewhat quicker than I expected. By the time I was facing 30, I had learned the biggest lesson of my twenties. And that was that life happens, and it doesn't necessarily follow the plan you had for it.

At the end of the decade, I was an "unmarried mother" and, although my anarchic side kind of relished being outside the circle of respectability, becoming a parent for the first time is always challenging, and it is doubly so when you do so on your own without the support of a partner.

I left the travel business I loved so much that it had become part of my DNA because the long hours and poor pay coupled with expensive childcare made it unsustainable. I could also no longer enjoy the delicious perks such as last-minute weekends in Majorca or the Canaries and wild "educational" visits to Mediterranean resorts, which were a huge part of why I loved the business. And although that was 35 years ago, so little has changed that my daughter has had to make the exact same choice in recent times. She worked in the travel business until baby number two made it unsustainable. Until working parents have a right to affordable childcare that is available to all, working women especially will have to change careers, sidestep promotions and generally lose out.

I think I also had a bit of an identity crisis. If I wasn't a travel agent, who or what was I? I wasn't married but wasn't quite single either. Being called an "unmarried mother" made me feel that I had failed at both becoming a mother and not becoming married. As my maternity leave came to an end, and I had to find a way back to work to support this gorgeous precious daughter and me, things got fairly dark and lonely.

On the other hand, there was a sense (and I put this down to the natural optimism of your twenties) that this was part of what women's liberation was all about.

Going it alone. Being able to do it all. Having it all. Who needed men anyway? Nope, not me. On a good day, I was determined to make all this work. To find a way forward for my daughter and me. But on a bad day, it was hard. Very hard.

Your experience of your twenties will not necessarily mirror mine. But I know from speaking to other women of our generation, many of whom didn't go to college and so began working in their teens and were married by their mid to late twenties, that it was the decade in which many of us grappled with adulthood. The freedom years did seem short, and if you weren't a single parent like me, you might have taken on a husband and a mortgage by the time you hit 30. I know one woman who describes waking up on the first morning of her honeymoon, looking at the snoring lump beside her and wondering, "Is this it?" Is this the view she could look forward to every morning for the rest of her life? Would it be enough? This beautifully expresses the shock of the reality check which often accompanied one's late twenties.

Many women of our generation had their first babies in their late twenties. And unless you are very, very lucky, this event will change your body forever. You may decide that your bikini days are over. Or maybe that is just me as I had an allergy to the relentlessly cheerful, upbeat physiotherapists who used to bounce into view while you lay in bed, still traumatised not only by the birth but by the fact that you were now a mother. They would cheerfully tell you about the importance of exercise to get your battered pelvic floor and saggy tummy back into shape. All of this while you were still worried about standing up in case all your innards fell through your now clearly enormous vagina.

Oh yes, your twenties will have been an interesting decade, full of new discoveries, new experiences, failed and successful relationships and the freedom that comes with adulthood.

But for women of my generation, it may also have been about losing that freedom again. For many of us, this was also the decade when life gave you the first kick in the shins, whether that be through heartbreak or, like me, finding yourself pregnant and alone. Some of our natural optimism and feeling of invincibility will likely have taken a knock in this decade.

By the time you are about to turn 30, you may well be a somewhat chastened woman. But there is one thing for sure, and that is that our twenties are formative years. It is during your twenties that you may well have first tasted how unfair life can be. How sometimes, just working hard or wanting something desperately is no guarantee of making something happen. Because all kinds of other things can come into play – things you never imagined could happen. It could be a broken heart, the death of someone close, an illness or any one of life's myriad of challenges. It is likely to be the first decade when you find yourself picking yourself up, dusting yourself down and carrying on.

We generally begin to lay down the foundations of our own resilience in our twenties. The first nuggets of wisdom are gathered, informing our opinions and choices, and we perhaps begin to realise that life is not always so easy.

# LOOK BACK AT YOUR TWENTIES...

**Self-criticism** – How did you feel about how you looked physically? Did you wish bits of you were different? Do you think this set up a pattern of self-criticism that may remain to one extent or another to this day?

**Hell-raising** – You might (or might not) enjoy recalling some of your drunken escapades as you grappled with alcohol in your twenties. A word of advice, though… never, ever share those stories with your teenage kids. Never. It's a massive parenting fail… and I know. I thought it was a great idea. I thought my kids would laugh and think I was great fun. Reader, they used my stories against me! You have been warned.

**Bad fashion choices** – If you "came of age" in the '70s or '80s will have great fun looking back at your fashion choices. The 1980s, in particular, was the decade that fashion forgot. We liked shiny fabric, huge shoulder pads and garish makeup. All of this coincided with a time when you are were figuring out your body and what fitted and what suited you. You might have fun trawling through old photos to see how "interesting" you looked in your twenties. And if you don't, your kids definitely will.

**Becoming an adult** – What were the things that happened in your twenties that made you realise, perhaps for the first time, that you were, in fact, an adult? What made you begin to accept the harsh truth that life isn't always a bowl of cherries? It could have been a bereavement, pregnancy, marriage, or mortgage. Do you remember moments when you thought, "Right, I'm a grown-up now, apparently"? Did one of the "becoming an adult" experiences make you lose some of the natural optimism of youth?

**How fearless were you**? – Did you challenge limitations put on you by parents, partners, work, colleagues, or society?

**How optimistic were you**? – Can you recall that glorious feeling that the world is very possibly actually your oyster?

Can you remember how it felt to realise that your parents were no longer really in charge of your life, but you were?

**Expectation vs reality** – As you began your twenties, what were your expectations and how did they pan out through the decade?

# THE TURBULENT THIRTIES

*"Calm her chaos but never silence her storm."*

**K Towne Jr**

## TURNING 30

Unlike my twentieth, my thirtieth birthday does stand out in my memory. Very clearly. It was the most tragic birthday ever. OK – so, no, no one died on my birthday. But I was a sad, lonely single parent who marked the beginning of my fourth decade on the planet by going to the local Chinese restaurant with my mother and two friends. The meal was fine, and I have a lovely mother and very sweet friends… but as a celebration, it was more appropriate for an elderly woman marking her eightieth than a mere slip of a thing marking her thirtieth. (OK, I was never a slip of a thing.) The truth was that I was excruciatingly lonely, and I was still coming to terms with how I had ended up somewhere I never expected or planned to.

I had assumed that I would be a successful career woman by my thirties with my own flat and car. I had thought I would be free to travel widely and regularly and that I would possibly be on the lookout for a serious relationship. I thought I would be deliciously free, independent, and professionally successful. However, as they say, life is what happens while you are busy making plans.

Becoming pregnant at 25 hadn't been part of my vision for life. Now, don't get me wrong. I always knew I wanted to be a mother. And in fact, it went further than that; when I visualised myself as a mother, it was always as a mother of girls. You might think as you read that "wow, she really did hate men", but I don't think that was the reason why I only saw myself with daughters. It was more to do with the fact that I grew up in a male-dominated household, and I had always wanted to have a sister. All my friends had sisters. And I felt that I had missed out on that experience. My friends probably wanted a dog or a cat. We had both of those, but I had no sister. Not even one. That is, I think, what drove my deep desire to have girls. So that I could experience sisterhood through them. It's a bit like a mother who dreams of a career on the stage but never makes it, so pushes her kids into stage school so that she can live her dreams vicariously through them. If I couldn't experience sisterhood myself, the next best thing was to watch it up close through my daughters.

By the time I turned 30, I had achieved my first daughter, albeit a bit early and without a useful partner… well, any partner at all. And so, although I was happy to be a mammy, I found myself marooned at home with my parents – not unusual nowadays but very unusual back then. As my friends were either married or well on their way to wedded bliss, I found myself in a kind of twilight zone of neither being as free as single friends nor married. I was kind of a spare wheel as all my best girlfriends were coupling up.

I had had to abandon my career in the travel business and now found myself working at something I didn't love (of which more anon). I wasn't in a great place. The worst part was that I couldn't see the future. For the first time in my life, I couldn't see the way ahead. I had always been able to visualise a future. I had always had a plan for the years ahead. But now I was becalmed in a dense fog with zero visibility and very aware that I was on my own.

Looking back now on that period, I realise that I was scared. I was scared of the huge responsibility for this precious young life I had mothered. I was unable to see how I could provide her with all I wanted to. It wasn't just that the future looked bleak; the future was invisible. I had no idea how I was going to manage. And I was lonely. Deeply lonely. Probably a lot more lonely than I realised at the time.

## NO EXPECTATIONS

Unlike my twenties which had sparkled invitingly ahead of me, my thirties stretched ahead like a dark, foreboding path through a dense forest on a cold, rainy night. I had no idea where I was going or who I could be.

I hadn't anticipated the difficulty I would experience in trying to keep my career in the travel business going while also being a good mother and father to my beloved daughter. Commuting into the city ate precious hours out of my day, and the low salaries in the business meant that paying for full-time childcare was also a huge burden. The perks of the job were now more or less out of my reach, as I couldn't head off to foreign shores at a moment's notice, one of the things I had loved most about the job. In order to shorten the commute, I moved company and began to work for a suburban travel agency nearer to where I lived. But the core issues remained. There was nothing for it, but I had to leave the business I loved.

As it happened, my dear mother rode to the rescue. She had recently begun her own business teaching word processing. Remember, this was 1988, and computer technology was still very new. Office workers were upskilling, and there was a huge demand for training.

So, it was my mother who suggested that I do a Teacher's Diploma in word-processing and join her. I felt I had very few options, so I did.

It was a lifesaver in terms of being able to work from home and tailor hours according to my daughter's needs. But I didn't enjoy it a whole lot. I liked the people, and so the teaching itself was quite enjoyable. I have always been a good communicator and my years of selling holidays meant I could sell anything. Well, I thought I could. And I have always loved a stage and an audience. But I constantly suffered from "imposter syndrome". I wasn't cut out for training this new technology, even if it was the most basic kind. I didn't find it interesting. I wasn't blown away by what computers could do. And most worrying of all, I was usually just a page or two of the manual ahead of my students. I lived those years in fear of being found out. I never was. Thankfully.

## THE STORIES

### *Women Are Phenomenal*

I learned the bare minimum I needed to about word-processing and computers during these years, but there was one lesson I learned that has coloured my life ever since, and that is that women are just bloody phenomenal. Mother's little computer training business offered one-to-one training and advertised mainly through local recruitment agencies. As a result, we got lots of referrals from these agencies. Many were women going back to work after taking a break to run their household and look after young children.

We discovered very early on that a shocking number of these women were being forced back into the workplace prematurely, usually as a result of a husband upping and leaving. These men were usually searching for their youth, which they thought existed in the arms of younger, childless women.

The women they left were often still in shock. First of all, they were often completely heartbroken. All of them had had their confidence severely knocked on all levels, and now there were often facing having to earn enough to cover the bills as their husbands, in some cases, had just completely cut and run. They were terrified of returning to office work which they knew was changing very fast with the introduction of computer technology. Workplaces were transformed worlds and had moved on a long way on from the golf ball typewriters they had left behind when they got married or had their first child.

We often called our clients "patients" because so many of them needed the time and space to cry and explain their fears before they could embark on learning the new skill they needed to get a job. Our office was our front room, equipped with two computers and a large box of tissues. We did sometimes wonder if we were doing the right thing by letting these women fall apart before we began helping them to negotiate this brave new world of computer applications. But we soon realised that they desperately needed to be listened to, to be heard. It didn't really matter what we said, but they needed to tell their story. And it wasn't always easy for them. Many felt mortified that they had been "abandoned" by their men. The shame they felt was tangible. We knew that in order for these women to have any chance, we had to help them find the confidence they would need to make progress. So, in many cases, the series of classes they had booked began with a talking session.

What I remember most about these women was their courage, strength, and unwavering commitment to their children. They were true warriors, wounded warriors but warriors nonetheless, who single-handedly managed to dress their deep wounds, put their families back together and not just carry on, but in many cases, to thrive.

I may not have learned much about computers, but I saw first-hand just how bloody amazing women are. Of course, all of this also served to reinforce my deep distrust and low opinion of men.

## Dating

In the end, living and working from home (although we did some onsite training, too) took a toll on me. I was deeply unhappy. I still couldn't see the future for my girl and me. I couldn't see how I would ever be able to provide for her in the way I wanted to, on my own. I was also very lonely.

I am not sure if it was because of, or in spite of, my man-hating that when my daughter was about 5 or 6, I began to date again. My opportunities to meet men were limited, as most of my friends were married by this stage; being a mother meant that I wasn't always free to go out, and I certainly wasn't up for very late nights when I had a young child with whom I shared a bedroom.

With the benefit of hindsight, I can now see that, along with seeking a meaningful relationship, I was looking for affection, for deep connection, and perhaps some kind of validation that my life wasn't over when it came to love. I was at my lowest point and made some awful decisions when it came to men. I did manage to find one or two very ropey boyfriends who didn't last long. My young daughter was a far better judge of men than I was and regularly objected loudly when introducing her to a new man. "Don't dare ever bring him to my school bake sale again", being one comment I remember flooring me. She was right. I didn't know what I was doing as I careered about, craving love, affection, and security in all the wrong places. I was in serious danger of walking myself into all kinds of trouble. I was all over the place. Then in one phone call, everything changed.

## Getting Over Myself

Our little training company regularly got calls from companies, usually former clients, looking to see if we had anyone on our books who might be suitable for a position, often an urgent short-term assignment. One of our clients was The Alzheimer Society of Ireland, at which I had trained the two secretaries in word-processing. A few weeks after completing their training, I got a phone call from the Chief Executive enquiring if we might have any suitable candidate for a temporary position as secretary, to cover some sick leave. We didn't, but I offered myself as a candidate without thinking as the conversation continued. We weren't busy at the time, and I was acting completely on impulse. I do remember I had to convince the CEO, who, for some reason, wasn't at all sure that I was a correct fit. He was a quiet man, and it could have been my aggressive selling of myself that caused him to hesitate. I was never backwards about coming forwards, and I think my experience of being an "unmarried mother" had certainly sharpened my edge. I was a bit of a bull in a china shop when I wanted something.

Anyway, long story short, a week or so later, I was working, temporarily, for one of Ireland's smallest and least known charities. I was the youngest member of staff by at least a decade, and the whole experience was a vastly different proposition to my previous job in the travel business, where everyone had been my age or just a wee bit older. But the people were lovely, and I was lucky to be working with a man who became the most wonderful mentor to me at a time when I really needed someone to give me back some sense of self-belief and confidence. Of course, I didn't realise just what a mentor he had been to me until much later.

Michael Coote was 80 years of age and the voluntary chairman of the society. He was one of the most creative, inventive, intelligent, and motivational people I have ever met. He saw something in me, and at the end of my temping stint, he offered me the newly created role of Public Relations Officer. I only had the vaguest clue as to what that meant, but if he thought I could do it, I was willing to give it a try.

I became a permanent member of staff in mid-September 1993. One of my first assignments in my new job was coordinating the visit of a contingent of cyclists from the UK who were doing a sponsored cycle on a 21-seater bike from Dublin to Cork to raise funds for the British Alzheimer Society. My job was to coordinate the press and media coverage and travel with the group.

To my 31-year-old self, this sounded as exciting as accompanying a pilgrimage to Lourdes (and I knew all about pilgrimages to Lourdes). So, moaning loudly to anyone who would listen, I set off one chilly October night to meet the ferry carrying this group of "anoraks from the UK and their daft bike". As I stood in the gloom at the ferry port, shivering in the damp air, the first person I met from the group was Paul Sherwood, the photographer with the trip.

He would be vital to my attempts to get media coverage and probably had much more experience with the press than I did, so I bounced over and introduced myself. Remember, I had never done anything like this before. He fell in love on the spot. Remember that I still pretty much-hated men. But he was a nice guy. I knew that.

The week on the road around Ireland went fine. The media coverage was great... thanks to the 21-seater bike.

When I came back, my dear girlfriends were all keen to know how I had got on. I mentioned Sherwood with absolute assurances that I was not interested. He was a nice fella but nothing doing. "But," they all roared "he has his own house and a good job". Seriously, what's not to fall in love with? I hated men. What can I say?

We stayed in touch, Sherwood and me. He invited me over to attend a reunion of the bike trip later that year. I stayed with him in his house, where he gave up his room for me because I had announced, "I don't do sleeping on sofas". Instead, he took the sofa. But still, I wasn't interested. And I was an outsize pain in the ass.

Sherwood and his sister, who had also been on the bike trip, came to Dublin for a weekend the following year, and I prepared a fabulous itinerary for them and accompanied them everywhere, but still, I wasn't interested. He definitely had the hots for me, which didn't help. I am a bit contrary. And I still hated men, although maybe not quite as much as before.

The following summer, I had booked a house in the middle of nowhere in West Cork (my spiritual home) to holiday for a week with my daughter. I was tired and felt the need to recharge in the peace and quiet of one of the most beautiful parts of the country. About a month before we were due to leave, I began to panic. At first, it was about the daughter. She was going to get bored on her own. My vision of reading books and just relaxing would not work if she was like a bag of cats. So, we roped in her best friend to come too. Then I began to panic about myself... stuck in the middle of nowhere with two kids, on my own. So, I asked a friend to join us. Then Sherwood phoned, and I asked him if he wanted to pop over too. The house had five bedrooms, and I suddenly decided to fill them. I asked another friend from the UK and his girlfriend to come too. So, this motley crew headed south for West Cork and a week in a little place near Clonakilty.

It was during that week, on a sunny day when Sherwood was pitched up against a tree in the garden reading a book (something which I now know he never does), that I realised that he was a lovely guy, kind, intelligent and most of all someone with a solid foundation, a sort of quiet inner strength that was very attractive.

I filed that thought, and at the end of our week in West Cork, knowing he had another week off work, I asked him if he wanted to accompany me on a week travelling around Cork and Kerry for work. And he did.

Our love story started in Dingle on the last night of that trip. In Benners Hotel.

We had been staying in B&B's as was appropriate when one is working for a charity. But on the last night, Sherwood insisted on booking us into a hotel, and so Benner's it was. In a room with a four-poster bed. He couldn't have planned it better if he had planned it.

We took the boat out to see Fungie, the erstwhile Dingle Dolphin, had a lovely dinner and a few drinks in a local pub and retired back to Benners. We ordered breakfast in bed for the following morning. All was well if you know what I mean, and we slept like babies. So much so that we were surprised when we woke up the following morning to find that our phone was ringing. It was reception to tell us that a waitress had been outside our door for ages knocking, and all she could hear was snoring. Our room service breakfast was now cold, but we were welcome to come down to the dining room. Which we did, sheepishly.

So, the lesson here, dear readers, is that snoring on a first date may not be a deal-breaker. Well, that is as long as you both snore.

## Finally... A Good Man.

In the end, I took a chance on Sherwood. My daughter, who was eight, approved immediately. This was obviously important to me, as it meant that he was clearly a huge improvement on some of my previous dalliances. I also decided that for a relationship to have a chance of success, I had to move out from home, where my inconsistent and often non-existent love life was a constant source of entertainment to my brothers.

So, I rented a little townhouse that I could only barely afford, and Sherwood began to "pop over" from Surrey every second weekend. He was an easy houseguest who happily washed up, cooked and was generally very useful. My cold heart was slowly beginning to... well, not exactly melt but certainly thaw a little.

I really liked having someone to tackle tasks that I would never dream of attempting – issues with my car, for example. I know, I can be really crap at feminism at times.

I drove a battered old Ford Fiesta called Bluey. I liked Bluey very much, but she had developed a problem with the window mechanism on the driver's door. Oh yes, we are talking windy up windows back in the early '90s. So, my window would wind down about a third of the way and then get stuck, making entering and exiting car parks a challenge. I usually had to open the door in order to reach the ticket machine. When Sherwood witnessed my hassle as we attempted to exit the car park at Dublin Airport, having collected him for the weekend, he decided that decisive action was needed and announced, "I will find a breakers yard tomorrow to get a used mechanism and fit it for you." God, I thought, isn't having a boyfriend just altogether wonderful.

True to his word, he found a second-hand window mechanism. On the Sunday, he set about dismantling my car door to replace the faulty mechanism. I played the dutiful girlfriend and made him coffee which I delivered to him out on the drive. I suddenly thought that being married might not be so bad after all. I could definitely see advantages.

Now Sherwood is not known for speed in anything he does. Slow and meticulous tends to be his modus operandi. So the sun was sinking in the sky when he finally announced that my car door was fixed and now had a fully functioning window. I was invited to come out and give it a try.

I was truly impressed as I got into the car, closed the door, and began to wind the window up and down. It worked a treat. "You are brilliant," I said, "just brilliant," and I was genuinely in awe of his ability to restore my car to its full functionality. Then I went to get out of the car. I couldn't. The driver's door was stuck. Stuck firm. But the window worked, which was in fairness what he had promised me. To get out of the car, I had to perform a deeply inelegant exit through the passenger door.

Sherwood was mortified. It was getting dark, and he was going home later that evening. When I saw him again two weeks later, we both had to enter the car through the passenger door, and he made the journey back to my place lying flat on his seat, which had eventually collapsed from all my clambering over it. But hey, the window still worked!

He is full of good intentions, so he is, but it's the execution of those intentions that sometimes falls short.

Some months later, he was washing up in the kitchen, and I was watching TV in the living room. He came in to me wearing a rather sheepish expression and brandishing my favourite coffee mug. You know, the one mug that makes your coffee taste just that little bit better than all the others. The one you MUST have your coffee in and into which tea should never, ever be poured. That mug.

He had the cherished mug in one hand and its handle in the other. "Em, it broke", he offered, "but I know it's your favourite, so I will superglue it back together." Now Sherwood is not exactly Bear Grylls, but he is rarely without superglue and a Stanley knife. No, I have no idea why. I am terrified of both, especially the superglue. Won't go near the stuff as I have visions of supergluing my fingers together and then having to go to the hospital to have the skin removed!

Anyway, once again, this drama unfolded on a Sunday evening, so as we left for the airport, my mug was sitting on the kitchen counter with its handle reattached. I was instructed to leave it there overnight to set but assured that I would once again be able to enjoy my coffee in its rightful mug in the morning.

Monday morning and freshly brewed coffee was ready. I went to get my mug which by now should be well set. And it was. Handle firmly back in place, and the mug glued solidly to the counter. And there it sat for another two weeks. A mini monument to my dearly beloved's DIY prowess.

I have a million of these stories because he never got much better at the DIY end of things. But at least we learned that if something expensive needs fixing, we find a professional to do it.

## Getting Hitched:

From that first get together snore-fest in Dingle, it took us only a matter of months to decide that this was it. Neither of us is particularly sentimental or romantic, but we are pragmatic. Back in the mid-'90s, being in your mid-thirties, certainly, in Ireland, it was considered a bit late to be getting married.

It felt a bit like waiting for the last bus, although you weren't sure you wanted to go home. A bus comes, and you get on, knowing that it's now or never. So, we both decided to jump on and became engaged at Christmas 1995, much to my father's relief and the bemusement of Sherwood's parents. I am sure they were somewhat nervous about their only son marrying a weird, loud, tall Irish woman who came complete with a nine-year-old daughter and whose mother had gifted their English son with a copy of the proclamation of the Irish Republic from The Easter Rising in 1916, to hang in his house. My mother has a very odd sense of humour. Although Sherwood is very sentimental about the proclamation, which still hangs in our hall.

Anyway, we were married in October 1996, back when weddings were merely a day out. My friends, like my dad, were delighted. On the other hand, my mother went off-road completely in her reaction to my getting married. She waited until the morning of the wedding to drop her bombshell advice. I was all set and ready to go. I had no bridesmaids. My mother was leaving the house with my daughter in one car; my dad and I were to follow in the bridal car a few minutes later. As I stood in the hall, she hugged me and said, "I wish you the very best of luck today. I don't think this marriage will last five minutes but enjoy it while it does." And with that, she left. I stood for some minutes slack-jawed, looking after her, waiting for her to come back and say, "ha, I am only joking. You and Sherwood will grow old together." But no. She didn't.

Now let me say that I wasn't upset by her words, but I was bemused. When I asked her about it later, years later, she said she had been practising reverse psychology. She maintains that I am a contrary daughter who doesn't do what is expected of me just to spite everyone. On that basis, she claims full credit for the fact that I am still married.

## Don't Call Me Mrs.

I just cannot write about being married without a rant about titles. Because how women are titled really, really grinds my gears. Let's begin with forms. Men get one choice, one box to tick. It says Mr Their marital status is of no consequence in their dealings.

By contrast, women find themselves confronted with three options on most forms. Mrs (which is usually listed first), Ms and most gobsmacking of all, there is often still a box marked Miss. Miss is how you address a girl. A child. It is the female equivalent of Master, but do we ever see Master on a form? Do we heck?

I remember the first time that this appalling imbalance struck me. I was in the local branch of a well-known opticians for the first time, and the guy behind the counter was filling in the form.

"Name?"

"Barbara Scully"

"Is that Mrs or Miss?"

"What?"

"Mrs or Miss?"

"What's that got to do with my eyesight?"

"What?"

"What has my marital status got to do with my eyesight?"

"Erm, what?"

"I am a woman if you need my gender. But my marital status is of no consequence."

The poor guy. He was covered in confusion and just left the 'title' box blank.

Surely the time has come for us just to be asked what gender we are so that we can choose to be male, female, fluid or neither.

And then there's Christmas. And Christmas cards. And every year, I lose my shit. Now don't get me wrong, I love getting Christmas cards. The problem is the envelopes they come in… or, more precisely, how they are addressed.

As you know, my husband's surname is Sherwood. I like his surname. In fact, I think his name is actually nicer than mine… but it's his. My name is Barbara Scully. I am not Sherwood because we are not related; we're only married.

Now I consider myself to be a tolerant woman, and I am fully aware that not all women share my view on this matter. I feel that true equality for women involves choice, but I am constantly amazed at how quickly most young women today rush to change their name after marriage. I think it's mad, but if that is what they want to do, that's fine. Good luck to them. My choice, however, did spare me the hassle of changing bank accounts, passports, and other legal documents.

In some countries, it is illegal for any person to change their surname without very good reason and marriage isn't one of them. Take Greece, for example. In 1983, feminist legislation included a law that all women must keep their own name after marriage. The province of Quebec in Canada has also outlawed women from taking their husbands' names since 1981.

Maybe we need a law like that here and in the UK. Then I wouldn't have to suffer the yearly ignominy of not having my name on the envelope some of our Christmas cards arrive in. The majority still arrive bearing the legend Barbara and Paul Sherwood. Or sometimes it's just Mr and Mrs Sherwood. Neither of which is correct. But every year, there is at least one which is addressed to Mr and Mrs Paul Sherwood – a form of address which airbrushes me out of the equation altogether. I am Barbara Scully. He is Paul Sherwood. All of us are the Sherwood Scully family. Is it that hard?

End of this particular rant.

## Mothering

When I was a little girl, I never dreamed about my wedding. I never imagined myself in a white dress "being a princess for a day". However, I always hoped that I would be a mother. Perhaps that was because I am lucky enough to have a great mother myself. So, my experience of the whole mother-child relationship was entirely positive.

I suppose it's not surprising that we have always had a great relationship, given my lack of sisters, something my mother also lacked. Come to think of it, my father had no sisters either. We are a family missing sisters having sisters.

## *My Mother:*

My mother Nor (short for Noirin) and I have always got on well, but when I was about 10 or 11 years of age, our relationship changed substantially when she decided that my cultural education needed attention. She still thinks I am a bit of a philistine, whereas she has always considered herself to be extremely erudite and a serious opera buff. None of this modern interpretation of classic operas for her. In fact, I don't think she even has much time for Gilbert and Sullivan, it being far too light for her taste.

Back in the 1950s, when she was a teenager, her idea of a great night out with her best friend was a night at the opera. Now, I remember how colourless Dublin was in the 1970s, so I imagine that in the 1950s, it was completely grey in terms of entertainment; but while the rest of the world was rocking around the clock in their blue suede shoes and the like, my Ma and her pal were hanging around the stage door of theatres to catch a glimpse of their operatic heroes.

Anyway, I had never shown any interest in her opera, probably because she was given to roaring various arias around my childhood home regularly. It scared the cats and put me right off opera forever. Even now, to my now reasonably cultured ear, opera still sounds too much like wailing for my liking, even when professionals do it. I know, I know. Maybe Nor is right, and I am a philistine.

However, she heard that there was a performance of Swan Lake coming to Dublin and thought a nice classical ballet would improve my cultural education, so she purchased two tickets and off we went. Now I will admit that I enjoyed it very much, although I don't think I have been to the ballet since. Did I say I was cultured? I may have lied! Much as I did enjoy it, I enjoyed the company of my mother more. And in fairness to Nor, she thought I was good company too. "We should do this more often," she said, and I agreed.

Opera was fairly thin on the ground in Dublin in the '70s; however, things took a turn for the better when the next performance she considered appropriate was much more to my liking. *Jesus Christ Superstar*, the rock opera, opened for the first time in Dublin in 1973.

Ireland in the '70s was still fiercely Catholic, and this rock opera was seen as quite outrageous. Some Catholics considered it blasphemous who protested its opening in a real-life forerunner of Father Ted's "down with this kind of thing". So at age 11, I knew it was pretty cool to be heading off to see the show, even with my mother. We both loved it.

Anyway, after Jesus came Joseph and his brothers and his coat of many colours and, due mainly to the fact that my mother fell in love with Pharoah, played by a singer called Cahir O'Doherty, we went to see this show every time it came to Dublin, which seemed to be every other month in the mid-'70s.

Mr Pharoah formed his own band, called wait for it… The Dazzle Band and so, although the cultural currency of the outings sank somewhat, my mother and I embarked on a remarkable odyssey around Dublin to wherever the band were playing. Taking one's 13-year-old daughter along to licensed cabaret venues to hear a showband would probably not be viewed as "parenting to aspire to" then or now. But for two happy years, we regularly got into her little Fiat 500 and chugged our way to all kinds of weird and wonderful venues in Dublin city and its outer suburbs. What my father made of this is unclear. And how much my mother told him of where we were off to is equally shrouded in mystery.

Of course, I was too young for these gigs, but I was never even questioned at the door due to the fact that I was heading towards my full height and, as I mentioned, great height induces all kinds of mad ideas, including the fact that you couldn't possibly be a child. We got to know the band, Paul Ashford, when on to play with another band called Stepaside, who were successful in Ireland in the early 1980s. So, a decade after the showband odyssey with my mother, my best friend Rita and I spent every Sunday evening at a Stepaside gig in Dublin. The fact that I was an old friend of the bassist and singer did me no harm whatsoever.

Those nights when I was 13, hanging around in smoky bars listening to old fashioned rock and roll with one of Ireland's last showbands, were exciting, and they certainly cemented a somewhat unique relationship with my mother. I didn't know any other girls who went out with their mothers, let alone to cabaret venues. I should also mention that my mother also bought me my first alcoholic drink around this time, a Babycham – a light and sparkling perry. The ad for it said, "Babycham sparkles, just the way I want to feel," and the logo included a doe-eyed Bambi. It was extremely innocent, although it seems creepy looking back now.

Through my teenage years and indeed beyond, there was little I didn't share with my mother. I entered my hippie phase immediately after I left school. Nor has always contended that the day I finished my final school exams, I had a sudden personality change, going from a steady, studious girl into a wilder, hippie-inspired teenager who was hell-bent on living all the life I missed during the years I was in school. I wanted to experience everything, drink everything and smoke everything too. I dabbled with hash regularly, and Nor got a little jealous. She had never been stoned and asked me to facilitate her experimentation by bringing her home a joint someday. Which I did. She was useless with it, as she had never smoked even a cigarette and couldn't inhale. I got more stoned than she did, and that was the end of her hippie phase.

Nor is one of the most non-judgmental people I have ever known. She accepts all her children's foibles, faux pas and major mistakes. Although I wouldn't like to give you the impression that she is above a good gossip. Because she is a great woman to have a gossip with. Always only indulge in gossip with someone you trust. Vital. And I trust my ma.

## Daughters and Sisters

I am the mother of three daughters. The eldest is married, a mother to my two wonderful grandchildren who live in Perth in Western Australia. As I write, my younger two are young adults and are currently in college.

As you know, our family started with me and my eldest. Then Sherwood, showing himself to be a much braver man than many people thought he was, joined us, and we had two more daughters. There are 12 years between the eldest and the middle child and less than two years between the middle one and the baby. The eldest was born in 1987 and the youngest in 2000.

I was nearly 39 when my youngest was born, and, from a physical point of view, both the pregnancy and the early years were much harder with her than when my eldest was born, and I was a young one of 25.

## Births

OK. Let's talk a bit about childbirth. Although it's painful, undignified, bloody, and messy, giving birth is a huge event in most women's lives. Each birth experience is carved into our very souls. Each birth changes us. Each birth I experienced was very different, although all took place in the same hospital.

## *Baby One: The Eldest*

As you know, I was a single parent. Back then, I living at home with my parents and two of my three brothers. My uncle also lived with us, as he had a learning disability. We were a very unusual family set-up, so I guess the fact that the eldest and only daughter was pregnant and alone probably fitted the profile.

My baby was due on the 3rd of August 1987, but on the night of the 27th of July, I started having what I assumed were contractions, although I wasn't sure, having refused to go to antenatal classes in case they frightened me. I still don't like to engage with stuff that scares me. Throughout the Coronavirus Pandemic, I avoided most news reports, daily statistics, and such. My middle name could be ostrich.

Anyway, back to 1987 and my "contractions". I decided it was best to wake my dear mother to enquire what a contraction felt like. "Jesus Christ, I can't remember," she said, which wasn't exactly helpful. Nevertheless, we both concluded that we should start preparing for a possible departure to the hospital. So, I had a shower, washed my hair, shaved my legs and had my mother paint my toenails. I was 25. These were my priorities. Although I was single. And you never know who one might meet in a hospital.

By about 1:30 am, we were making plans to leave. One of my brothers was sober (the other one had just got in from the pub and was most definitely not, and the third one was away), so he decided he was in charge of operations. My mother was getting herself into a bit of a spin which made her giddy and not particularly helpful. Meanwhile, my father stood at the top of the stairs, like a lighthouse perched on a high rock as he silently viewed all the kerfuffle in the hall below. Me? Well, I was shell-shocked, I guess, at the realisation that I was probably about to become a mother. I felt more than a little wobbly with a heady mix of blind fear and excitement.

As I picked up my hospital bag, which was by the front door, my "man in charge" brother yelled orders at us, "Barbara, you go in the front. Ma and Jim, ye are in the back". My father rather nervously asked, "em, should I come too?" "No room for you, Da, go back to bed," said he in charge, ushering us all out into the night towards the yellow Renault 4 on the drive. As we all piled in, I suddenly remembered something a good friend, who was already a mother, had said to me a few weeks earlier when she was worried that I was being too much of an ostrich about the impending birth. "You will have lovely new nighties for your confinement," she had said, "but make sure to bring an old one for the birth." Now, this pronouncement had prompted immediate visions of an abattoir, so I had buried it in the back of mind. But now, it surfaced, like a cork in the ocean, as I faced the prospect of actually giving birth.

"Wait", I cried. "I need an old nightie. I haven't got one in my bag".

"No worries," said mother. "I'll run in and grab one. I have one I haven't even worn yet, but you can have it."

A few minutes later, we took off, my brother driving as fast as the old banger of a Renault 4 would go. As we rattled and shook our way towards the maternity hospital, we raced amber traffic lights, squeaking through junctions as I hung on to the passenger door, which had been known to fly open when the speedometer reached 30mph or more.

Then I realised that my "contractions" had stopped. "Right," I announced. "I feel fine now. Let's go home. I am not in labour. False alarm. Home please, I want to go back to bed."

"Oh no," said brother in charge. "I am not going to have you delivering this baby at home or on the side of the road. No, no, no. We will take you to the hospital and see what they say."

"But, but… I want to go home."

Despite this, we roared into the hospital grounds and rumbled to a halt at the front door where the car was abandoned, and we all tumbled into the reception area, which was manned by a night porter. I was still protesting loudly.

"Are you in a hurry, Mrs? 'Cos if so, you go on, and your husband here can give me the details", he said, looking at the brother in charge.

"He's not my husband, he's my brother and NO, I am not in a hurry. Take as long as you want." The night porter made no more assumptions after that, poor man.

Form filling completed, we took the lift to the third floor where we were met by a bemused night nurse, who asked us to keep the noise down. I explained that I was here against my will, that my contractions had stopped and that I wanted to go home.

But the nurse was from the same school as my bossy brother. "Well let's see about that. In you go, put on your nightie and I will give you an examination. We will probably keep you in overnight anyway. The posse you brought with you can go home."

I was glad to bid them all farewell as I pulled the curtain around the cubicle and rummaged in my bag for the nightdress my mother had loaned me.

As I pulled out what I knew was one of her infamous "remnant" creations, my heart sank. Once she found a piece of fabric she liked for half nothing (and she liked lots of clashing colours and big designs), she bore it proudly home, like a cat who had unexpectedly caught a fabulous exotic bird in the garden. Then she dug out the old Singer sewing machine and, without a pattern and, I'm convinced, often without even cutting, she would fashion (and I use the term lightly) a garment for herself. This nightie was one of her creations.

It was a simple design – two armholes and an empire line which was outlined in that Ziggy Zaggy stuff which was de rigueur in the 1970s. Bear in mind, however, that this was 1987. I put my head in the neck, tried to get my arms through the armholes and got completely stuck. Afraid that the nurse or, worse still, the doctor (this is before women doctors were really invented) would barge in at any moment, I forced my arms through, ripping it down both sides. Then I went to pull it down over my bump. I pulled, and I pulled. It covered the bump, but it didn't really cover my bum. To this day – 30 years later – I don't know why I didn't just get one of my fabulous new nighties out of the bag and abandon my mother's creation.

But I guess it did make it easy for the nurse to give me "an internal" and establish that I wasn't in labour yet. Apparently, I had experienced some 'Braxton Hicks' – a term I hadn't heard of, because of my avoidance of prenatal classes. But, true to her word, the nurse put me to bed where I lay awake most of the night listening to the snoring of the woman in the next bed who had given birth that night.

At the first sign of activity on the ward the next morning, I requested permission to leave. I needed to get out before my mother had phoned all and sundry, telling them I had "gone in". This would mean facing the very public humiliation of a false alarm. However, I was under doctor's orders, and he hadn't surfaced yet to make the call on whether I qualified for parole.

In the end, I got so agitated, they phoned him, and the decision was made, that since I was there, he might as well induce me; save me the bother of going home and having to come back in a week or so – which was when my baby was actually due.

I had no idea what induction involved. But it began with an enema and having my waters broken, neither of which I would relish experiencing again. I seemed to have spent an hour or more on the toilet and was convinced I was going to deliver my poor baby into the murky pan. Enemas are now a thing of the past. Thankfully. Then I was attached to a drip and told to get walking.

It didn't take long before I realised what contractions really felt like… at which point I was moved into the delivery room. Being partner-less and husband-less, I was on my own, and, as I was dealing with the epidural and bracing myself for what was ahead, the midwife announced that my mother had arrived. "Will I bring her in?" she asked.

"No. Do not. Tell her to go home. We will call her when there's news."

Now, this might seem a bit heartless, but I knew that if my lovely, slightly mad mammy arrived in the delivery room, I would give up all involvement in this birth and start to cry, just like one of those young ones on *One Born Every Minute*.

In the end, my baby arrived at 3:30pm. This baby girl I had known forever. And the one that changed my life utterly. As she was placed back in my arms, after being checked and measured, and before the nurse had a chance to phone home for me, she said, "oh, and your mother left a huge bouquet of pink flowers."

To this day, I don't know how she knew, but she did. But that's my ma for you.

## Baby Two: The Middle One

By October 1998, I was Mrs Respectable. Pregnant again, but this time with rings on my fingers and a husband at my side. Now, one of the unforeseen disadvantages of being a single mother first is that one tends to have heightened expectations of childbirth and pregnancy with a partner.

I was working full time, so I would arrive home exhausted every day by my third trimester. I would manage after a little snooze to get through dinner but would generally be in bed by 10pm at the latest.

As I have already mentioned, himself is a good man and tries his best to be thoughtful but sometimes doesn't quite manage the join the dots. One day, early in my third trimester, he arrived home, delighted with himself, telling me he had bought me a present. I only had a few minutes to enjoy the anticipation of a fabulous massage oil, or some aromatherapy bath bombs, or maybe just a fab moisturiser before he brandished a concert ticket under my nose. "I got us tickets to see Paul Young at Midnight at the Olympia."

I looked at him, wondering for a moment if this was a joke. I mean, I had liked Paul Young two decades earlier. But a gig at midnight. "Sherwood, I haven't seen midnight for weeks," I answered, trying to keep the exasperation from my voice. "There is no way I am staying up until the early hours, even for Paul Young. Sorry. Thanks, and all but no thanks." Sherwood managed to look like how I imagine Babycham Bambi might look if someone kicked him in the gob. But he wasn't going to let his ticket to waste. So, off he went on his tod at about 10:30pm to head into the city. I went to bed. I was, however, gracious enough to wake up when he returned. "How was it?" I mumbled.

"Paul Young was grand. But I think I might have hit a fox on the road on the way in, so I was a bit upset and couldn't really enjoy it."

It turned out that he had been so upset he had driven to the cop shop and handed himself in. Even though the fox had run off. Once the gardai established he wasn't drunk, they let him go. But the night wasn't what anyone could call a great success.

Then there was the time that I was so exhausted when I came home from work that I took to the sofa for a nap. Sherwood was very understanding. He has always been a great believer in naps. As he cosied me with a blanket, I asked him if he would just make our bed, having remembered I had stripped it that morning. "Sure," he said, "you relax and sleep." And so, I did. I woke an hour or so later and hoped that I might smell food being prepared as it was gone dinnertime. Nothing. No lights on either. Darkness had descended. In fact, no sign of Sherwood anywhere.

I went upstairs to change, and yep, there he was. In bed. Asleep. AND HE HADN'T EVEN MADE THE BED FIRST. That time we had a row. I couldn't believe it. I was so sure that having a husband would mean I would be pampered and attended to through my pregnancy. I called a friend. "He's useless," I cried down the phone. "I want a proper husband who will mind me." "He is a proper husband," this wise friend said, "but when you are pregnant, it's your mammy you want because they get it. Men really don't."

So true. I reigned in my expectations after that and curbed my disappointments.

Baby number two was due in mid-November, so I went on maternity leave at the end of October. Then on the 30th of October, I did it again. I went into false labour. Off we went to the same hospital, to be told again that I wasn't really in labour. I was told to go for a long walk around the grounds and returned later. After two laps of the grounds, I decided I was hungry and wanted McDonald's. And so off we went to the local drive-through and ate our Big Macs and fries in the car. After that, I decided we would go home. I was mortified that I still didn't know what labour was.

However, in the middle of that night, I woke up to go to the bathroom, and as I stepped over a sleeping cat on the landing, my waters ruptured. The cat got a terrible fright and was a bit wet. Sherwood called Nor to come over and babysit the 12-year-old, as off we went to the hospital for the second time in 24 hours.

This time I had left it a bit late. Labour was well established, so I was told I was too late for an epidural. Bad news for Scully. But all went well, and by sunrise, our Halloween baby had arrived into the world.

The thing I remember most about her birth is the feeling afterwards. Perhaps it was because no drugs were involved, but I experienced the most incredible high, which lasted for weeks afterwards. I felt like Queen of the World. A goddess who was powerful beyond belief.

This euphoria caused me to cut short my maternity leave, so, at 8 weeks old, my precious baby went to creche, and I went back to work. I regret that to this day. It was stupid. I don't know what I was trying to prove and to whom I was trying to prove it. But I figured it was to do with being superwoman – giving birth and returning to work in jig time. Stupid. Stupid. Stupid.

## Baby Three: The Baby.

So, as many women will testify, when your baby is about a year old, many women experience an intense urge to "go again". I was no different, and although I had a teenager, a baby and a full-time job, I desperately wanted to have another baby.

Sherwood was aghast. Then again, he had never really wanted babies in the first place. I think that was part of my attraction to him. I had one who was half-reared already. On the other hand, he didn't know he wanted cats either until he met me.

Anyway, I convinced him that I didn't want the middle daughter to be like an eldest daughter who had essentially spent most of her childhood as an only child. We went everywhere with a pal in tow for her. So, it made sense to make our own pal this time. He finally agreed; this third pregnancy would also be my last.

I was approaching 40, and my body was not quite as keen on the pregnancy lark as it had been previously. I put on loads of weight and my ankles, a cause for grave concern for all who knew me. I waddled merrily into work every day, but I felt more than exhausted by 6pm when I was leaving the office. Often my car was parked at the top of the road I worked on, which was a hill, and I regularly wondered if I would manage to make it to the top without requiring oxygen.

Baby three was due in November, but by early September, I felt totally exhausted all the time and, like millions of mothers before me, I wished that this was over and was dreading the last weeks. Well, as the saying goes, be careful what you wish for.

On the night of the 14th of September 2000, I went to bed early, but I woke up at about 2am, feeling distinctly uncomfortable and wet. Yep, my waters had broken again, but this time I was hoping that this was all a dream. After about 20 minutes, I realised that I probably needed to wake himself and put in the call to Nor to come and babysit as we took off into the night to the hospital.

I clearly remember the cold fear that this was too early for my baby to be born. I still had six weeks to go in my pregnancy. She was born quickly, and when I was told that she weighed in at an impressive 8lbs 12ozs, I felt confident that her prematurity would not matter one bit – wasn't she well ready for the world?

However, an hour after her arrival, the paediatrician came to visit me and, with a grave face, told me that our infant girl had severe breathing difficulties. This was because her underdeveloped lungs could not support her sturdy size. She was in special care, and the next 48 hours would be critical. We were taken down to the unit to see her. Nothing could have prepared me for seeing my new, beloved little baby lying, strapped down in the incubator with tubes and monitors covering her little body. This precious gift of a perfect baby girl was in imminent danger of being taken away, and I couldn't do anything. Worse than that, I couldn't hold her. I couldn't comfort her. I couldn't whisper in her ear that it would be OK. I couldn't make her better.

Once I was over the initial shock, I resolved to be strong. I didn't want to cause unnecessary worry to the other members of the family, who I knew would take their cue from me. I made a point of telling everyone I could that our baby was very ill and asking them to pray and to send her healing and love. I spent as much time as I could in the unit, gazing in at her and sending her all my love and strength through the Perspex wall of her incubator.

Early on her third morning, I made my way to the unit to see how she was – 48 hours were about to elapse – were there signs of her coming on? Things were not good – her temperature was up, and the nurses feared he had an infection, which could be very bad news indeed. They were setting up an X-ray to investigate, and the paediatrician was on his way. My baby was crying. I stood helplessly by the side of her glass box, and I cried too. I have never felt more helpless in my life. I felt I was failing my daughter. What could I do? Absolutely nothing. I was also in the way. I made my way back to my room.

As I looked out the window at the rush hour traffic, I wondered how people could be going about their daily lives when I was looking into an abyss. I was on the brink of a place so dark I could not imagine how I would survive if I was to have to visit it. I phoned my husband and tried to be honest without making him feel as bleak as I did.

I went back to the Special Care Unit – they were still working on my baby. I turned around and headed back down the corridor, my heart growing cold. Without thinking about where I was going, I found myself down in the oratory of the hospital. I would not regard myself as religious, but I do pray. When life gets tough, really tough, I find that praying gives me something to do. But I also believe that my prayers carry power, whether that is out to the universe or to some being like a God, I don't know. But I pray. I talk to God, Mary, Angels, and goddess Brigid. I try to cover all bases.

As I sat in the oratory and stared at the single lit candle on the altar, I began some serious negotiations with God. I promised to give up everything that, up to this minute, I had thought was important if she would just get my baby through this crisis.

I would resign from my job and look after her myself. I promised I would be the best mother I could be if she could just pull through. My arms ached to hold her. My heart was broken from being separated from her by the transparent box in which she was lying. I closed my eyes and realised that what I wanted more than anything was to be at home. At home in our little house with my other two daughters, my husband, and this new baby safe and tucked up in her Moses basket in the corner. I held this vision in my head and willed it to happen as I made my way back to my room.

I slept and dreamed of dressing her in pretty babygrows and tucking her up in fluffy white blankets.

When I woke, I immediately returned to the Special Care Unit. She was sleeping, and all activity had ceased. The nurse said that the tests hadn't shown anything and that her temperature seemed to be coming back down. She suggested that I should try to express some milk so that, if she kept improving, they might try feeding her some through one of the tubes. Glad to be able to do something that felt vaguely useful, I went to acquaint myself with the milking machine!

Baby seemed to be peaceful all through the rest of that day. She seemed to be concentrating all her energies, too, into becoming stronger. I spent hours sitting beside her, continuing my conversations with God. That night I couldn't sleep and at about 1am, I padded down the corridor again to see how she was doing. The night nurse said that her temperature was back to normal, and she had just given her some of my milk through her tube. For the first time in three days, I felt that there was finally mothering my new baby. I felt there was finally a real physical connection between us. I blew her a kiss goodnight, and sending thanks heavenward, I returned to bed.

The next day, all her stats had returned to normal. She was still being helped with her breathing and being monitored very carefully, but the paediatrician felt that she had turned the corner. I was now allowed to open the little door on the incubator's side and hold her little finger. We spent hours touching hands, and still, I whispered her encouragement to get strong.

I remember all the milestones of the final days in Special Care from this point on. On the fourth day, the nurse took her out of the incubator, and I was able to hold her for a couple of minutes. I cried with the joy of finally being able to hold my precious baby. It was the most precious gift I could have been given. The day I had to leave the hospital, my baby was taken out of the incubator, and I could at last dress her in the pretty babygrows that were waiting for her. I visited twice a day on her final four days in the hospital. The day before she came home, it was time for her to have a bath. Would I like to do this, the nurse asked?

Would I ever? As I bathed her carefully in the tepid soapy water, I finally thanked God out loud for the normality of it all.

Each baby changed me and my life in reasonably major ways. I have written already about being a single mother. My middle baby reawakened some latent power in me, which gave me the strength to cope with the terrifying first weeks of my youngest daughter's life. And in the aftermath of the fright I got and given the knowledge she would have some health issues relating to her breathing for her first few years, I began to consider changing all our lives in a major way.

I was contemplating taking just a year off work in order to spend time with my baby and tend to her needs. I had a dream of a domestically blissful year; I imagined days in the kitchen in a haze of flour wrapped in a fug of baking as we made buns and chocolate cakes. Autumn walks, even in the rain, afternoons collecting shells on the beach, or in the park feeding the ducks; coming home to light the fire and while away another hour colouring-in and drawing. We would be poorer but content. Safe and happy in our domestic bliss. And Sherwood was entirely on board with this plan.

But for the moment, there was still work to be done, and one day in September, just before my baby's first birthday, I was involved in making an offsite company presentation. Afterwards, I made my way back to the office feeling relieved and happy that it had gone well. I was still nurturing my dream of a gentler life just beyond the horizon. Oh yes, God was in her heaven, and all was right with the world.

This was before the days of smartphones and social media, so in my bubble of contentment, I casually wandered back into the office and was surprised to find my colleagues gathered around a TV in the boardroom in utter silence. I stared at the screen, trying to make sense of what I was seeing. A plane had crashed into the World Trade Center. It was a beautifully clear, blue-sky morning in New York. "It can't have been an airliner. It must have been a small private jet," I offered because an airliner couldn't just crash into the World Trade Centre. And then, as we watched live on Sky News, just after 2pm, a second plane hit the other tower.

A knot of fear and dread formed in my stomach as the realisation dawned that this was no tragic accident.

I stood, petrified by the atrocity that was happening, live on air, in a city that is so familiar. And it just kept getting more horrific. People jumping to their deaths, and then the towers collapsing, taking with them the lives of so many more, including firefighters and police. The world seemed to be tipping slightly off its axis as these images burned themselves deep into my brain, where they still live.

On the 14th of September, Ireland held a national day of mourning. All shops and businesses were closed. The following day was my baby's first birthday, and I had no card.

The world was still engulfed in the news from New York. I tried to shield my youngest two from the replaying horror as it seeped from the radio, TV, and newspapers. My dream of an idyllic, gentle, domestic life that I had for so long held in my head, and my heart suddenly seemed to be built on very shaky foundations. Then my three-year-old drew a picture of the towers on fire, and I cried at the contamination of innocence.

The following January, I bid goodbye to my thirties.

# THE WISDOM TAKEAWAYS.

Even if you manage, unlike me, to sail happily through your "golden twenties", free as a bird, living life large, loving, travelling, and working, the thirties is a different ball game altogether. It is the "is this it" decade. The decade you finally learn that you can't control everything.

It is most likely in your thirties that some part of your grand plan for your life will start to fall apart, whether that's a relationship or lack of one, children or lack of them, or a career stall. Or you may have already had a kick in the shins in your twenties, but it's in your thirties that many of us finally begin to seriously grow up.

Through my work, I know many young women who are now in their thirties. Back when I was in my thirties, many women were dealing with that question of 'is this it?' as they coped with marriage and lots of small kids. By contrast, I know many women now spend their thirties looking for that relationship and worrying about having children as they work hard and forge the career they will need to fund the things they ultimately want. Not massive luxuries but a roof over their heads that is warm and comfortable.

In many ways, life was simpler for my generation, although also, in other ways, it was harder. Perhaps we were more pragmatic when it came to choosing life partners, or maybe that was just me. But we were probably the last generation who could hope to pay a mortgage and raise kids on one salary, which is generally not possible today. This makes life much more complicated for women as they climb the career ladder with their biological clock ticking louder in their ear with every year that passes. Gender equality still has some way to go in creating a world where women and men have equal opportunities not only for career advancement but also for caring for and raising a family. Because, from where I sit, the burden of trying to combine both still falls unfairly on women.

My thirties were, yet again, a decade of two halves, just like my twenties. The second half of my twenties was me trying to cope with being an "unmarried mother". That coping and struggling continued into the first half of my thirties, and it is one of the defining experiences not just of my twenties and thirties but of my life.

Life as a single parent led me to run straight into the wall of patriarchy, bringing down shame and guilt on my head. I realised just how hard society's norms are to push against. My self-esteem took a battering, which led to a pretty dark period. That darkness meant that, for the first time ever, I couldn't see the way ahead. I couldn't see my future, which was very frightening.

It was also the decade when women's strength was fully illuminated to me. Working with and talking to the women who were valiantly trying to put their lives back together after a separation made me realise the depth of women's reserves of courage. We never know just how strong we are until we are truly tested. Women have an inner strength that makes us phenomenal. All of us.

My thirties also taught me that life can change in a couple of minutes. For me, it was that one phone call that brought a job offer. That, in turn, led to me meeting the man I am still married to and two more daughters. Although it's only with the benefit of hindsight that you can pinpoint the moment of change.

Hindsight also allows me to say that, although I became a mother in my twenties, albeit not in a planned way, I can now see that it was in my thirties when I fully embraced the power of being a mother. Childbirth is a privilege, but it's also part of what makes us so strong. Louise Erdrich said, "*women are strong, strong, terribly strong. We don't know how strong until we are pushing out our babies. We are too often treated like babies having babies when we should be in training, like acolytes, novices to high priesthood, like serious applicants for the space program*".

Becoming a mother also made me fully appreciate the fact that I had been mothered by a remarkable woman myself. And I know that makes me lucky. I know that being biologically related to someone doesn't guarantee anything.

This was the decade that also taught me that family is everything for me. This is something I didn't fully understand until my youngest daughter's premature arrival into the world and the fright I got when there was a chance that she wouldn't make it. That made me realise that life is sometimes very simple. A warm, comfortable home, supportive partner, and my children (and my four-leggeds) is all. Everything else is just window dressing. The icing on a cake. Nice icing. Nice window dressing and enjoyable too. But just added extras all the same.

By the end of my thirties, I was in a very different place from where I had been at the end of my twenties. I was a "respectable" (eyes north), married woman with three kids, a job I loved, a mortgage and my own cats. It seemed like I finally had it all. Just as feminism had promised. Look at me, I thought. I am Wonder Woman. I did it. I have it all.

It should have felt so exciting. But it didn't. It mainly felt exhausting.

# LOOK BACK AT YOUR THIRTIES

**Marriage** – Did you get hitched? How did that feel? Or perhaps you always assumed you would marry but ended your thirties without it happening. How did that feel?

**Motherhood** – Did you become a mother in your thirties? How did the birth(s) change you? Did you feel magnificent or maligned? I know some women who found childbirth (for a myriad of reasons) to be quite traumatising.

**Your mother** – Did becoming a mother cause you to reflect on how you were mothered? How is your relationship with your mother?

**Fertility** – Did you struggle with fertility in your thirties?

**Career** – Did you have a paid job? Were you progressing in it as you had hoped to?

**Is this it?** –Our thirties is often the decade when we wake up to the fact that perhaps life hasn't exactly turned out as we had planned it to as a teenager or in our twenties.

It is often in our thirties that we begin to wonder, "Is this it?"; 'is this how my life is going to be?' Did you think that?

**Expectation vs reality** – As you began your thirties, what were your expectations and how did they pan out through the decade?

# THE ROARING FORTIES

*"Sometimes we don't want to feel like a postmodern, postfeminist, over stretched woman but rather a Domestic Goddess, trailing nutmeggy fumes of baking pie in our languorous wake."*

**Nigella Lawson**

## TURNING 40

When I turned 40 in January 2002, I thought it was time to celebrate. I wanted to banish the ghosts of my sad thirtieth "celebration" a decade earlier. I was in a good place, busy and happy. The Celtic Tiger was beginning to stalk the land, which meant that we all felt more abundant than we actually were. It was time to throw a party. A proper party, much like my 18th, in a hotel, with a DJ and food, only this time the guests wouldn't have to pay to attend. And so I did. And it was grand. The new decade suitably marked and celebrated.

I felt more in control of my life than I had a decade earlier. But at times, it did feel like it was teetering on a cliff edge with chaos below. The eldest was 15, and we had a toddler and a baby. I had a full-time job, and he was working for himself, which usually meant very long hours. Life was busy. Very busy. I was juggling it all and felt like I was dancing backwards while doing it. It was very exhausting.

I loved my job and had thought I could do it all. But the truth was that I couldn't. Well, I could… just about. But it wasn't merely hard work. It was extraordinarily stressful. Increasingly I felt that I was a drunk juggler praying every day that, when I dropped a plate, it wouldn't break. "Having it all" really does mean doing it all.

These were the "hurry up" years. They were the words I seemed to use most often with my kids.

"Hurry up and eat your breakfast..."

"Hurray up and brush your teeth…"

"Hurry up into the car…"

"Hurry up the steps into the crèche…"

I was always hurrying up, always feeling like I was pushing a rope up a hill, and yet always being behind schedule. Every day I arrived at my office, somewhat frayed and bedraggled, feeling like I had already done a day's work. These were the years of driving home with babies in the car, talking and singing like a maniac so that they wouldn't fall asleep, which would destroy the evening altogether. The years of washing breakfast dishes as I prepared their dinner, of falling asleep while reading them a bedtime story. The years of hanging out washing on the line at 9pm and sometimes having my dinner at 10pm. Having it all, my ass.

The relentlessness of all the pressure was crushing. And it was the source of many tensions between myself and himself. Neither of us had nine to five jobs, and that added an extra layer of complication to the juggling. There were regular arguments over whose job would take precedence when we discovered we had both committed to working the same evening. Usually, I capitulated as I didn't get paid overtime, whereas Sherwood had clients to keep happy. It was really crazy. And I remember clearly the day we both woke up to just how crazy and how unsustainable it was. We had arranged to rendezvous in the city because we needed to swap vehicles. He had a commercial for his work, and I had the family car with the baby seats. And, as I was working late, he was on duty to collect from the crèche, but that meant we had to change vehicles. With the cars bumped up on a footpath, we stood in the rain swapping keys on a dark winter's night, and I remember saying to him, "this is fucking nuts." I think that was the moment I woke up and decided we couldn't do this anymore. My youngest still had some lingering health issues wise related to her prematurity. Things began to feel increasing "wrong". I began to wonder about our quality of life. I had a feeling that something had to change.

Sherwood had first suggested that maybe I should consider taking that year out to settle everything down and regain some perspective. Just a year, I thought. I could do that. In twelve months, I thought, I'll be back at work. Because I was still, in my heart, a career woman. (Why I wonder, is there no such thing as a career man?) And wouldn't I go mad in the head altogether if I were at home all the time with just my own kids for company?.

So in the last months of my thirties, I had retired from the world of paid work, pausing a working life that had spanned 22 years, to dive into that unknown life of a "housewife". I cried bitter tears as I packed up my desk at work, took my photos off the noticeboard and walked out the door for the last time. However, by the time I got to my car, I could feel a burden lifting. Because the guilt I had experienced working full time while I had small kids had been smothering. I also knew that we were about to take a huge financial risk to indulge the dream of a calmer life – and, dare I say, a better life.

I had that new vision of myself as a kind of domestic goddess, running a home, baking cakes, cooking delicious and nutritious meals, being very hands-on with the kids while he went out every day to bring home the bacon. Yeah, I know, I can hear you say (again) – "I thought you were a feminist?" I did wonder if I was selling out, letting the sisterhood down. But that only makes sense if you think that the role of full-time homemaker/housewife/childcarer is not valid work. I had learned, the hard way, that for me, it was actually the most important work I could be doing when my kids were small. And I had also learned that having a partner to share the labour of earning the money and running the home and kids works best if it is done equally. It's up to you and your partner how you work that out. And I know I was lucky. Due to the booming Irish economy, Sherwood was completely free of any domestic responsibilities so that he could work all the hours he could to make the money we needed. Meanwhile, I looked after everything else.

This arrangement may not work for everyone, but it absolutely worked for us.

## GODDESS EXPECTATIONS

So, as I turned 40, the pace of my life had slowed considerably. The mania of the juggle had stopped. I could now focus on home and kids. I felt like an explorer leaving my tent after a wild storm and finally being able to survey my surroundings.

Shortly after my new life began, on a cold winter day, a former colleague phoned me in the mid-afternoon. I was out walking, pushing the double buggy around our local village. I remember telling her that I was out for a walk with both my youngest kids and I had a lasagne cooking in the oven that would be ready when I got home. In that moment, I knew that, despite having walked away from a job I loved, I was doing what I was meant to be doing. The stress had lifted. In fact, I was enjoying my days in a way I hadn't in years. But more than all that, I felt like I was back in control of my life, in as much as any of us ever really are.

One of my first priorities in this new life was to fix the preparation of food, which had been so scattergun while I was working full-time. A "by the way" here --when I refer to 'working full-time', I mean outside the home for a salary that is paid into my account every month. I cannot say "outside the home" each time I say working because that would be so irritating. However, you can assume that that's what I mean. But let's be clear. I very much think that running a home, with all that involves, and doing all the childcare and domestic chores is a real job. Just because it is not paid, not valued by anyone except the family it benefits, has no defined coffee, lunch, or even loo breaks, does not mean that it is not legitimate work. It most certainly is work, and it is worthy, worthwhile, skilled and comes with a huge responsibility.

OK, where was I?

Food. I have described previously how having kids in daycare and working full-time meant that by the time I got home every evening – often near 7pm, my priority was to get the kids fed and into a bath, then begin the process of getting them to bed. I am a little ashamed to admit that I didn't spend the weekend batch cooking meals that I could serve easily during the week. So, the food most evenings was pretty "convenient", and that is a way of avoiding saying, not particularly nutritious. There were a lot of fish fingers and chicken nuggets. By the time the kids had gone to bed, I was completely exhausted, and I will admit that we ate take-outs more than we should have. Not every day clearly... but often more than once a week.

So, giving up work meant that I could up my game on the meal front. The girls weren't as relieved and pleased as Sherwood was. He just loved coming home to a proper homemade meal, and we managed to all eat together more, too. Win, win.

Preparing home-cooked meals was one thing, but what I really wanted to do to qualify as a domestic goddess was to learn to bake. And no, I wasn't influenced. This was long before *The Great British Bake Off*.

Oh yes, my forties were going to be spent in domestic bliss, making memories with my children, getting more cats and baking a few times a week so that, whenever anyone called, I would have some delicious confection to offer them, and my kitchen would permanently be wrapped in a warm, yeasty aroma. I was upbeat. I was confident. Ireland was flying. The economy was booming, and all was well in the world! And so were we. Sherwood and I found that our separate roles suited us very well.

Around this time, I also discovered that I cared less about what people thought about me. I felt able to take chances again, possibly for the first time since my teens or early twenties. I started writing. I had my first article published. A full-page in a national Sunday paper – it was such a thrill.

I finally felt like an adult. Mortgage, check. Kids, check. Cats, check. Part-time writer, check. I felt grown up. I was no longer a girl. I was finally a woman. And I found I had the time to ponder some of the things that being a woman involved.

Oh yes, I am a woman. Hear me roar.

# THE STORIES

## Married Money

One of the first things that struck me about our new working and living arrangement was that I needed to amend my views on money. Just because we had chosen for me to stay home, where I couldn't earn any money, didn't mean that I should feel powerless or dependent on Sherwood. We were a team. An equal team. In everything, including our finances.

There has long been a tradition of women having their "running away money" in Ireland. This goes back to the days when women were barred from working after marriage. Although, even if a bar didn't exist, it was generally seen as a slight on one's husband if a married woman worked. Women who wanted to work were told that they were disrespecting their husband by so doing, as they were signalling to the world that they had no confidence in his ability to look after his family financially. This kind of nonsense was not just confined to the fifties housewife. Oh no, these attitudes continued right up into the 70s and early 80s.

Women who had no access to their own finances often secretly squirrelled away money every week, money they skimmed off their housekeeping allowance, which was their only source of income. I remember my Dad handing Nor (my mother) her housekeeping money every week. Women were keenly aware of their complete dependence on their husbands. The house and bank accounts were in his name, giving him complete control over their lives. So, I fully understand why women needed to have a safety net in the form of a small nest egg they could access alone. Known as 'their running away money', I am sure that many women used it for just that, women who may have been in dire circumstances otherwise.

However, those days are over. Along with more rights, we have ATMs and electronic banking. So, one thing that I think women of all ages should wise up on is sharing all resources within a committed relationship, including money. When we decided that I should confine my energy to the home front while Sherwood went out to work, it was agreed that the money he earned was not his money. It was our money. And I had equal access to all the accounts, just as I had when I was bringing home equal earnings to him. If you love someone enough to embark on a mortgage and, more importantly, have kids together, then surely you should trust each other enough to share all the financial resources too. No more "running away" money unless you are in dire circumstances – in which case all rules of this kind are out the window as women should do what they need to to survive.

## *Periods*

Back in 2013, a story hit the news about a Russian lawmaker who asked his parliament to consider allowing women two days of paid leave every month when they menstruated. The Russian was quoted as saying, "during their period of menstruation, most women experience psychological and physiological discomfort." He went on to say that, in some cases, women are so discommoded they require an ambulance. This rather over-egged the pudding and detracted from his argument somewhat, I thought.

Needless to say, any comments I saw in response to the Russian lawmaker were entirely dismissive of his suggestion, which was regarded as sexist and silly. The implication was that women were not in any way put out by the arrival of the monthly bleed. Periods are a breeze. Ever since the invention of tampons, we can even go swimming and horse-riding, cheerfully wearing white trousers while bleeding. And sure, with a reasonable supply of Solpadeine or Nurofen, you don't feel a thing. Right? Because admitting that periods often make you feel really crappy is letting the sisterhood down, right? That would be a sign of weakness, a sign that we are... well, less macho than the guys. Right?

Around the same time, Bodyform, the manufacturer of feminine hygiene products (sanitary towel maker in other words), decided to address a Facebook post by a Richard Neil, who sought to expose the lies contained in the advertising of feminine hygiene products. Richard wrote the following on the Bodyform Facebook page (reproduced exactly)...

*Hi, as a man, I must ask why you have lied to us for all these years. As a child I watched your advertisements with interest as to how at this wonderful time of the month that the female gets to enjoy so many things, I felt a little jealous. I mean bike riding, rollercoasters, dancing, parachuting, why couldn't I get to enjoy this time of joy and 'blue water' and wings!! Damn my penis!! Then I got a girlfriend, was so happy and couldn't wait for this joyous adventurous time of the month to happen ....you lied!! There was no joy, no extreme sports, no blue water spilling over wings and no rocking soundtrack oh no no. Instead I had to fight against every male urge I had to resist screaming wooaaahhhhh bodddyyyyyyfooorrrmmm bodyformed for youuuuuuu as my lady changed from the loving, gentle, normal skin coloured lady to the little girl from the exorcist with added venom and extra 360 degree head spin. Thanks for setting me up for a fall bodyform, you crafty bugger.*

Bodyform apparently thought Richard had a point and, in an ad they posted on YouTube, Caroline Williams, fictional CEO, admitted that their ads had lied, but made the point that their focus groups in the 80s couldn't handle the truth of periods, with mood swings, cramps and so on. She even referred to "crimson landslides".

I can understand why Bodyform and other similar manufacturers might lie about periods – they have a product to sell. But are we, modern women of the 21st century, living in the so-called first world also lying – to each other and to our girls about periods?

In 2006, BBC2 screened a series of programmes called Tribal Wives. In each episode, a different British woman went to live for a period (yep, I did that on purpose) of weeks with a 'primitive' tribe in various parts of the developing world.

One particular episode stands out in my memory because it dealt with what happened when that week's British woman got her period. In the tribe, menstruating women had to go to a special hut on the outskirts of the village. So, off our British woman went, somewhat horrified that she was being "put out" of the village as if she was unclean. But she found the experience to be very soothing. In the special hut, she was minded by other women who braided her hair, and she was not expected to do any work. After a few days, she returned to her duties in the village feeling refreshed.

The novel, *The Red Tent* by Anita Diamant tells the story of Dinah, daughter of Jacob, one of the infamous 12 sons, one of whom supposedly had a multi-coloured Dreamcoat.

Dinah grew up with many mothers, as Jacob had multiple wives. As is generally the case when women live together, their menstrual cycles synchronised, so the Red Tent was where the women of the extended family went while they bled. For three days and nights, they did no work, no cooking, but spent what sounded like a reasonably relaxing time chilling out together in their own female tent.

As I read the part of the book that described the actual red tent, I found myself being ridiculously envious of these Old Testament women and their special "time out" place.

I am old enough to remember when sanitary pads and tampons were only ever advertised in women's magazines. In fact, when I first started menstruating, my dear mother arrived with the most enormous pad you could imagine, safety pins and a belt of knicker elastic. The belt was worn around the waist, and the pad had a loop on each end with which to secure it with pins to the belt. I put it all in place and, as I lolloped around, I found myself muttering, "get off your horse and drink your milk." Pads with sticky backs, although still huge, were a marked improvement. As for tampons... well, sure, that was just brilliant. Once you got used to where to put them. Remember, I had no sisters and Nor seemed to be behind the curve with her belted pads, so I relied on my friends' advice as I tried to orientate my 13-year-old self with this foreign part of my body.

Over the last few years, there has been a campaign around period poverty in Ireland and elsewhere. In fact, the topic was addressed by a young female TD in our parliament. And you know what I am going to say next, right? Yep, if men had periods, not only would the working month only have three weeks, but all sanitary products would be free and delivered to your door every month. It is truly appalling in this day and age that women and girls living in poverty can't get tampons and pads when they need them.

I digress. But seriously, sisters isn't it time to stop pretending that we don't bleed and admit we sometimes bleed a lot every month. Isn't it time we stopped pretending that periods are a breeze? Periods are an intrinsic part of being female, but they can make you feel crap. Cramps, sore breasts, feeling bloated, having to carry a handbag (because we often don't get pockets on our clothes either) and being near enough to a decent loo every couple of hours are just some of the monthly tribulations.

Surely it's time for us to reclaim ALL it means to be female. But sometimes, just sometimes, like maybe once a month, wouldn't it be wonderful to have a special tent full of comfy sofas and beds and pillows and – for those that wanted them – scented candles and soft lighting and chocolate? Just think about that.

Of course. A uterus also needs regular maintenance once we have been sexually active, which means a regular smear test. And oh, what fun that can be.

## Having A Smear

At the outset, let me categorically state that I believe in the absolute necessity of regular smear tests. I have twice had precancerous cells detected that required further treatment, and I am glad to say that my smears have been normal for the last number of years. But my history means that I am called every year for a new test. So, I consider myself a bit of an expert.

I was probably twenty-something when I took myself off for my first ever smear. Our family GP back then was a lovely chap. He was a tall, angular man in the mode of Basil Fawlty, with a mid-Irish Sea accent and an easy laugh. Being a woman of the world, I thought, "I am not going to seek out a female GP who I have never met before. I can do this with your man I always go to".

So, the appointment was made, and I presented myself at the surgery. His greeting to me was always the same "Oh Barbara, oh good. How are you?" "Hi Doc," I answered, trying to calm the butterflies in my stomach, "I am here for a smear test". His face displayed that rare combination of delight and puzzlement. "Oh right. A smear test you say. Great. Golly gosh no one has come to me for a smear test in years. I normally just see all the old women round here."

My heart sank, and my brain roared, "mistake Scully, big mistake." He ushered me towards the bed with the usual instructions to remove all my lower garments and said he'd be back in a minute. To this day, I suspect he consulted some medical manual to remind himself where he was likely to find my cervix. Minutes passed as I lay there until I finally heard him re-enter the room, and his face came around the curtain wearing a big grin and what looked like a miner's lamp strapped to his forehead. "Jolly good, we're all set," he announced, as he blinded me with his "headlight". That test took ages, but it was "jolly good fun" by all accounts.

The following years, my gynaecologist carried out my smear tests due to a combination of recent childbirth and my odd cells. But some years later, I was back at my local GP.

Basil Fawlty had retired, so my current GP was a younger man. But it seemed that all the other women in the village knew what I still did not. *Go to the practice nurse for a smear test.* So, although he wasn't quite as gleeful at the prospect of furkling around in my undercarriage, he was just as at sea. "Right, you get sorted there and shout when you are ready," he instructed as he pulled the curtain around the bed. I took off my shoes and looked around for a modesty blanket.

"Erm, where's the blanket, Doc?"

"What blanket?"

"The blanket. I am not going to lie here with everything on show. I need a blanket".

"Oh, right. Back in a minute."

So once again, I lay there while he went off in search of a blanket.

Finally, he returned, and an arm came through the curtain brandishing a blanket. A picnic blanket. A very small one. A scratchy one. "Please tell me you didn't get this from the boot of your car", I pleaded. By now, he was right grumpy. "No, I didn't", he barked. So, I disported myself on the bed, knickerless, looking like I was wearing a tartan mini skirt a la Vivienne Westwood at the height of the punk era. In the distance, there was the sound of a penny dropping.

The following year I made an appointment with the practice nurse. The room was nice and warm. There was a gorgeous soft yellow blanket, and she was that wonderful "nursey" combination of common sense and empathy. As she approached with KY Jelly in one hand and the speculum in the other, she announced that she was using a plastic implement. "More comfortable, and not as cold", she assured me. Everything was going reasonably smoothly as she began her furkling. "Oh, I think you have a tilted cervix", she muttered with only a small hint of exasperation. Then a loud crack, like a gunshot, rang through the surgery. It emanated from my nether regions.

I nearly fell off the bed with the shock. I am sure some elderly patients in the next-door waiting room got a right fright too. The nurse turned a bright shade of red. "Well, I have never had that happen before," she said as she retrieved her speculum, which was now in two separate pieces.

So, the moral of the story is – go to the practice nurse for smear tests and beware of plastic implements.

## Magic Knickers

By my forties, having given birth to three children, I had abandoned all thoughts of getting my girly figure back again with all its shortcomings. But I felt I could do with a little help, and who should come along with just what I needed but those two wagons, Trinny and Susannah and their magic knickers. Magic knickers were guaranteed to lift your bum hold in your tum and were designed to stretch up all the way to just under your boobs. I couldn't wait to get my hands on a pair. I know I paid a fortune for my first pair, purchased in a proper lingerie shop.

It was Christmas, and we met some friends for a posh dinner. I excitedly pulled on my magic knickers and my new festive outfit and took a look in the mirror. Definite improvement – a lot of the lumps and bumps had magically vanished. "God Bless Trinny and Susannah," I thought, and off we went. It was as we were walking into the restaurant, waving at our friends who were already seated, that I had the very disconcerting feeling of my magic knickers magically rolling themselves back up as though their job was done. Like my school tights, I think my magic drawers had been designed for shorter women. I spent an uncomfortable night looking lumpier than ever as my own excess poundage came up for air, joined by a redundant roll of expensive undergarment.

Of course, things have improved since the early days of the magic knickers, but "shapewear" is still making all kinds of promises that are rarely delivered.

I will admit that it took me well into my fifties to realise that there really isn't a painless and non-invasive way to make a flabby belly disappear. Because I decided magic knickers weren't for me, I again splashed out on a different undergarment that promised to pull me and suck things up to where they wouldn't cause offence. I had a fancy awards ceremony to go to, so I bought... no, I invested in a "body" corset yoke with shoulder straps, so it couldn't fall down. It had poppers underneath for ease of peeing and seemed to be exactly what I was looking for. And just like the magic knickers, things went well initially. I definitely looked a little more svelte in my long dress. It was a great night which involved quite a bit of wine. Then I had to visit the bathroom. Have you ever tried to refasten poppers in your undercarriage in a small loo cubicle while intoxicated? I nearly contorted myself into a serious injury. And no, I am not of the generation who could bounce out of my stall to seek the help of other women, whether they may be known to me or not. I was gone so long and came back with a face so red that my dearly beloved was highly suspicious as to what I was up to. Until I told him.

As you would expect, after its first outing, I washed my expensive undergarment, put it in the dryer then put it away for its next big night out. I thought if I drank less, it might be easier to manage. Another fancy do, and I was being picked up by taxi. As I bent over in my attempt to elegantly fold my six-foot frame into the car and not trip over my long dress, there was a faint popping noise, and a breeze whistled past my nethers. Yep, my body (the corset one, not the physical one) had obviously shrunk. I was late, and it would have taken too long to undress completely to remove my underwear, so I just carried on. It wasn't an altogether unpleasant sensation once I got used to it. And it did make peeing much easier.

## Reality Bites

2008 had been a great year for us, but things started to change towards the autumn. I was 46, our youngest was 8, the middle one was 10 and the eldest turned 21. He was busy, and I had begun to write seriously and had my first pieces accepted for radio broadcast, earning proper money for the first time in a decade. We took our first holiday to the USA that summer, and in September, I decided to spend my radio earnings (with his blessing) on a cookery weekend with a friend in Italy – and yes, radio paid way better back then than it does now. Italy was sublime; however, I do remember chatting at the airport about the crash of Lehman Brothers in New York because, according to the news reports, this could potentially be very serious. Although I must admit that neither my friend nor I had any real understanding of how it could be serious and weren't particularly worried about its effect on our little damp island in northern Europe.

By the time autumn had truly arrived, things had indeed become very serious. The economy in Ireland was beginning to collapse. We kept thinking it would be a short-lived crisis that would soon be over. But instead, it kept getting worse and worse, month after month. Two years later, my husband's business was seriously struggling. We had begun to save a few years earlier, and we had also started a fund for our kids' college education, but by 2010 we had no reserves left. It was all gone, and by Christmas of that year, we were barely hanging on.

Every month was a real challenge. He drastically cut his fees as he chased down every lead and did some jobs which were hardly worth doing for the amount he got paid. We cut our living expenses down to the bone. Every week I pushed my trolley around the supermarket, trying to tot up my spend as I went and stopping when the money ran out, regardless of what we still needed.

Ireland was on the brink of a bailout when I wrote this (slightly edited) for the Irish Times, encapsulating where we were.

*It didn't look like a Black Thursday. September 30th 2010 in Dublin was a lovely mild day with blue skies littered with a scattering of white clouds. No breeze and just the slightest hint of autumn in the air. It was a day when you should be glad to be alive. A day when the earth was trying her best to distract us with her beauty and benign nature.*

*On Twitter, others noticed the beauty of the day too and the platform was alive with photos of a sparkling Dublin City. As Morning Ireland came on air, Twitter began discussing the current state of affairs.*

*There was a building sense of seriousness. The jokey tone of a couple of weeks ago was gone. The main feeling was one of disbelief. I continued to scroll, reading each comment. In 140 characters (as it was then) there is nowhere to hide. No room for flowery language. Twitter tells it like it is.*

*I phoned my husband, who was already out chasing up work, and told him not to turn on the news. Tune your radio away from talk and listen to rock music all day, I commanded. As a self-employed sole trader, he has more than enough on his plate wondering about paying next month's mortgage. He didn't need to know about another harsh budget in December. Not today anyway.*

*As I hung up the phone, I began to get angry. I am a housewife and part-time writer. I have no degree in economics or politics. I don't understand bond markets. But I am not stupid. I run a home, write, support my husband's business, and raise our children. I am a citizen of this country. My opinion counts. And I am angry.*

I was angry, really angry about lots of things. Angry with the ineffective government who let things get to the stage they did. Angry with the subsequent government whose measures crucified so many less well-off families while allowing the wealthy to make ever more money as they picked over the fire sale of assets and property.

I was angry that I had to watch my husband run himself ragged trying to keep earning enough to keep our boat afloat and our bills paid. And I was angry that there were so many other families in similar situations or worse all over the country.

It was a horrible time.

We still look back at those bleak years and wonder how we survived. It wasn't just the anger but the fear and dread we both felt all the time. That knot in your stomach as you wake up each day and wonder what bad news the day will bring. The dread of something breaking down, such as the washing machine, and knowing you won't have the money to replace or repair it. Taxes went up, and new taxes were introduced, and each time we looked at each other and wondered how we would manage.

I remember chatting with some friends who were all in their late forties/early fifties like us. We were all broke, and some were very worried about their jobs. We were all exhausted from just getting by with an applecart that was just one apple away from disaster. And none of us had ever expected to be under such stress about money at that stage in our lives.

And yes, I know we were the lucky ones. Many families lost more than their savings and peace of mind; they lost their homes. The fact that, over a decade later, we still have thousands of children without a place to call home is deeply shocking and shameful.

The economic collapse wasn't just a temporary blip but an earthquake that left everything utterly changed.

My husband probably paid the highest price. He developed prostate cancer in 2016, and I am convinced that the huge burden of stress he carried through those years played a large part in his ill-health. But there was one good thing to come out of these dark years. Something that has worked for us ever since. It is my job to be up when he is down and vice versa (and this is most definitely not a euphemism). On his dark days, my role is to bring light and hope. And he does the same for me. Those recession years broke us in every way except emotionally. It cemented our teamwork, which, as it turned out, was just as well.

# THE WISDOM TAKEAWAYS

So, in many ways, my forties, much like my twenties and thirties, were another tale of two halves. We roared along very happily, with the decade panning out much as I had anticipated until the roaring turned to bawling as the Celtic Tiger upped and left the country, and we wondered how we would manage to stay afloat financially. It seems that the universe taught me not to take stuff for granted. I was still learning that nothing stays the same for very long. Still learning to really enjoy the good periods because something totally unanticipated and totally outside of your control can come out of left field and change everything.

It was the decade that began with my realising that working full-time while also trying to run a home with young children is not only stressful but for me (and many women, I would imagine), there was a bucket load of guilt that came with it. I could normally keep that guilt suppressed until something went wrong. The mornings when my small baby had a temperature or gummy eyes (conjunctivitis), meaning the creche was out, were always days when I had an important presentation to make or a vital meeting to attend. The guilt of negotiating and juggling to make it to sports days and nativity plays was huge. And I was lucky, as I worked only a few miles from home and school, but it was still stressful. Because I knew where I wanted to be, and it wasn't at my desk or making a presentation. It was minding my sick baby; it was watching my little one being a wise man or angel or coming last in the class race on Sports Day.

I was lucky. And for once, my timing was bang on, so we could make the choice for me to leave the world of paid work to discover, much to my surprise, that I loved being at home with my kids and running our home. But I also learned just how much of a job being a "housewife" is. Women who stay at home contribute hugely to our society but do so silently and invisibly. (And I know there are some "house husbands", but it is still mainly women.) Perhaps in our rush for equality, we have raced ahead, demanding, quite rightly, to be paid the same as men and to be given the same opportunities, but we have forgotten the sisters for whom running a home and raising children is a job: a hugely important job. In our rush to abandon "traditional gender behaviour models", have we denigrated a role that many women (and men) believe is their most important one – that of homemaker?

Being at home with children is only possible when you have a partner who sees the role as equally important to his/hers, which is to earn the money to keep the show on the road. It's truly a team game!

But how many of us "housewives/house husbands" have been asked when we are going back to work, the implication being that we clearly aren't working when we are running a home and caring for kids. How many of us experienced that dilemma of finding an appropriate answer to the question of "what do you do"? We struggle to justify our lives in the home.

We have silenced this army of stay-at-home parents. They work away within their homes, volunteer in their communities, run residents' associations, and make endless cups of tea at school events they have most likely organised. These parents are working and are contributing to society. We do not value their contribution half as much as we should.

Equality for women is all about choice. And yet I know many women who feel they have let down the sisterhood by abandoning their education and career, albeit temporarily, to care for their offspring. Women continue to struggle to live in a world that has been created by men for men, who mostly had wives at home looking after the domestics and the kids. I don't believe we will ever have true equality until we dismantle and totally redesign the world of work. We need far more than affordable, high-quality childcare, preferably near our workplaces; we also need far more family-friendly flexible work practices. The entire culture around work needs to change. Some of that change may have started thanks to the Covid-19 pandemic, which forced companies to immediately facilitate working from home, proving that change can happen far quicker than it usually does.

Shortly after I morphed from PRO to Domestic Goddess, the brilliant broadcaster Gerry Ryan did an item on the radio about women in the home and how they are not appreciated. I wrote in and was invited on air. We chatted for ages on the topic, and he got me to admit (on national radio) something that I hadn't really realised until he asked me directly about it. His question was about when I had been working how I had felt about women who didn't return to work after their first baby was born? I said that I had thought they were taking the easy option. By the time I admitted this to the nation, I knew I was wrong. Very wrong.

I had discovered that women will never achieve equality until the work of caring is properly valued. I include in this all carers and those who work in the care industry and are paid so badly. Feminism's next job is to address society's attitude to this hugely important work. And this is why we need a lot more women in politics and in boardrooms so that we have a critical mass of female input into decision making. We need to change the world to one designed for families and where the work of caring is at the very core of a much healthier society.

During my time at home, I also learned how important it is to have full transparency and honesty around money. Once you stop earning your own salary, you become totally dependent on your partner's income. But we were very clear in the months when we were considering this huge change in our lives that, if I was to be at home, my contribution to all our lives would be just as important as the money he brought home. I was not going to be made feel that in some way I was sponging off him because without me at home, he wouldn't have been able to work without spending huge amounts on childcare and domestic help. The money he earned was our money, and I had just the same access to it as I had had when I was contributing half of it.

Speaking of money, I think it is fair to say that the world's economy and especially Ireland may not have crashed so dramatically and fallen into such a catastrophic recession if we had more women where it counted. I have no doubt there would have been less risk-taking in our banks and more compassion deployed in our government strategy for recovery.

However, for our family and with the benefit of hindsight, this whole episode taught us to take nothing for granted. By the time I was coming up to my fiftieth birthday, I knew that change was upon us again. I was beginning to understand just how lucky I was to have had that lovely decade at home with my children. We were lucky that I left my paid job just as the economy was taking off, so Sherwood, working long hours, could earn enough to keep our boat afloat. I cooked, baked, walked on the beach with the kids, and we got a dog. But I honestly believe that all families should be facilitated in having one parent at home, especially while there are pre-school children in the family. And yes, that means that they should be paid. It should not be a privilege to parent your own kids. It should be a choice. A legitimate choice offered to all families.

So, everything was pretty great until it all fell apart. And although, by the time I was coming to the end of my forties, we were in a far more precarious position financially than ever before, I knew that we just needed to hold on, to keep going, because, as that old saying goes, nothing stays the same for very long.

# LOOK BACK AT YOUR FORTIES

**Having it all** – If you are a mother, you will probably have discovered that "having it all" is nonsense in your thirties or forties. It usually means nothing more than doing it all. How did that work for you if you had a paid job and young children? And how did it make you feel? Or perhaps you did manage to "have it all".

**Working mom guilt** – Most women I know suffered from this when balancing all the competing demands of family and a job. Did you experience WMG?

**Domestic goddes** – Did you harbour dreams (perhaps secretly) of becoming a domestic goddess, being Queen of your kitchen, running a home that looked fab, smelt amazing with the best-behaved kids and animals imaginable? Or was that just me? And if it was you too, did it work for you?

**Caring with no reward** – If you decided to take time out from paid work to care for your children, how did that work out for you? How did you feel when someone asked you what you did? How did you describe yourself? Do you think society puts value on the work of caring?

**Being a woman** – So, in your fourth decade of dealing with the joys that female biology brings with it, what are your thoughts on periods and how we cope with them? Do we need to be more open and vocal about what a nightmare it can all be? What do you think of the idea of Red Tents? I'm serious!

**Other people's opinions** – It's often in our forties that we begin to stop caring quite so much about what other people think of us, of how we look and of our life choices. Did you experience that in your forties? And if you did, did you find it liberating?

**Expectation vs reality** – as you began your forties, what were your expectations and how did they pan out through the decade?

# THE FABULOUS FIFTIES

*"You're not getting older; you're getting more entitled to be your fabulous self."*

**Gwen Stefani**

## TURNING 50

There is no doubt about it - turning 50 is a big deal. It is probably one of the most anticipated birthdays of all, right up there with your 21st. It feels like a huge milestone. But it is a somewhat sobering birthday. You have probably passed the halfway point of your life. You have less road ahead of you than what you have left behind. Naturally, this realisation prompts some soul searching on what you have achieved or done and what lies ahead.

As I cruised towards the big 50, I was convinced the meaning of life would somehow suddenly reveal itself to me. I waited and waited for this revelation to write something deep and meaningful. I waited for the wisdom of age to arrive. Frustratingly, it never did. I sat down numerous times in the hope of writing wise words that would surely come easily with this great age. They never did.

At this point, I must say more about my friend Rita, who I mentioned briefly earlier; she has been involved in every big birthday celebration since I was a girl. Rita is my oldest and one of my closest friends. We met when we were seven and have been friends ever since. We now live across the road from each other.

The weird thing is that we are exactly the same age, born on the 11th of January 1962 – her at home in suburban Dublin and me in Holles Street Hospital in the city. So, we have celebrated all the big milestones together, although Rita isn't a show-off like me and so has been happy to attend my parties while having her own more elegant and private celebrations. Our lives have many parallels which are more than a bit spooky. We both have three kids. We both lost a sibling. We have both had gall bladder issues and had our respective gall bladders out within months of each other by the same surgeon.

I mention Rita now because she managed to develop a strategy on her fiftieth birthday, which was a lot wiser than my self-indulgent navel-gazing. She said that once she reached 50, she would always have a bottle of champagne in the fridge. She wouldn't be keeping it for major celebrations either. She would crack it open whenever she felt like it. She was always a bit of a devil with the drink, but I think this was the wisest thing I heard from anyone about turning 50. It's a more polite version of Helen Mirren's wishing she had said 'fuck off' more as a younger woman. And it's great knowing your pal across the road always has chilled champagne and is willing to open it at the drop of a hat.

As me and Rita hit 50 in January 2012, the country was still gripped by recession. So it was never on the cards for me to have another big party. In fact, there wasn't even a small party. But there was something that I had a desperate urge to do.

In June the previous year, my eldest, like hundreds of thousands of Ireland's young people, had decided to emigrate. Emigration is something of a way of life for the Irish. I think as a nation, we carry some kind of wanderlust gene that makes us extremely curious about the world beyond our shores in a way that few other nationalities do. This wanderlust and openness to travelling is also one of the first ways we confront disaster, especially when we are young. Irish people have been emigrating for centuries. So, in the face of a failing economy and the lack of jobs, our young people again took flight in huge numbers. They went to Canada, to the UK, and, as with my eldest daughter and her boyfriend, they headed south to Australia.

Of course, she didn't announce she was leaving to find a new life elsewhere, somewhere she and her boyfriend (now husband) might find more opportunities than were on offer in our bankrupt little country. No, she began talking about taking a year out of life to travel and see a bit of the world. Although there did seem to be an awful lot of research going on into Australia. However, I was distracted with everything going on and didn't really pay attention until the day I was racing out the door as she and her boyfriend were sitting at the kitchen table, and she casually said, "Just booking our flights to Perth, Ma."

I was on my way to collect one of her sisters from football, and I remember asking her to wait until I came home before doing anything. As I drove towards the football pitch that evening, I finally accepted what I had been avoiding for months. My eldest, my firstborn, my precious baby girl, was leaving Ireland. I was heartbroken, but I knew, from that moment, that it was the right thing for her to do. And I knew that in her shoes, I most likely would have done the very same thing. And so it was that on the 6th of June 2011, Barbara Scully, aged 49 and a half, along with himself and the other two, said goodbye to our eldest. "It'll just be a year, Ma," she said, but she was crying too.

While emigration is a big part of life in Ireland, it is a surreal experience. The day she left, we were all bereft. Although her visa was only for two years, I think we all knew that this was one of those huge days that would change all our lives forever. As a parent, the pain of the emigration of one of your children is not unlike bereavement. OK, so no one is dead and with today's technology, the separation is not as complete as before. But knowing her voice and face is only a click away is not the same; not the same at all as being in the same space, being able to touch her face, and smell her shampoo. In the months after she left, there were days when I was so angry that I couldn't just be with her, having a coffee, or lunch or just a laugh. Nothing beats being around someone's energy, especially when you love that someone with all your heart. So as I approached my fiftieth birthday, I only wanted one thing: to go to Perth.

Instead of presents, I sought donations to my travel fund because I was going to mark this new decade by travelling halfway around the world to a country I had never, up until that point, had any real curiosity about. I would mark my big 50 with a trip to Perth to see my girl and her new life. But what I really wanted was just to sit and have lunch and a chat with her. I wanted to look into her eyes because only then would I know for sure if she was genuinely happy with her new life. I suspected that she had fallen in love with this new city and country. I also needed to see if it was deserving of her affection.

In the end, we all went on a trip made possible by the arrival of the first of the Middle Eastern airlines to Dublin, bringing lower fares. We have always prioritised travel. When other families might be buying a fabulous telly or great sofa, we would use whatever disposable money we had to travel, especially when there was good value to be had. And those introductory airfares to the other side of the world were relatively reasonable.

So, we all got to see our girl. And we came to understand why she had landed where she did. Western Australia is a special place, and Perth is a beautiful city on the water. But more than that, I got to see her life close up. And travelling to Perth is something I have continued to do regularly – well, until bloody COVID-19 I did. I know my daughter's local supermarket almost as well as I know my own, which makes me happy. Perth is like a second home now, and it makes the 14,000km that separates us feel a bit less of a distance.

## REINVENTION EXPECTATIONS

Turning 50 is a big milestone. It can be a sobering transition into the second half of your life. It is a time when you look back over the decades and wonder about your life. For women, especially if you have kids, turning 50 can also mark the beginning of an evolution. You are keenly aware that your kids are getting older and more independent. They need you less and less. And whether you worked outside the home or not, this is a huge change in a mother's life. There is freedom beckoning from just over the hill.

However, as I began to contemplate this freedom, I was also aware that we were still in the teeth of a recession. Money was still an issue. I needed to go back to paid work and start bringing in, if not a side of bacon, at least a few rashers.

Contemplating going back to work after a decade spent out of the workforce is terrifying enough but knowing that you are now classed as an "older" woman only adds to the terror. It, of course, shouldn't be like this, but it most definitely is.

I knew that getting a job was going to be very difficult. There weren't many opportunities on offer, to begin with. But I also soon realised that being 50 and having spent a decade "at home" weren't attractive traits to potential employers who clearly thought I had spent those "lost years" lying on my sofa, eating chocolate and watching daytime TV.

I began my job search by visiting the local employment office, where two perfect jobs involved writing. I enquired at the desk, only to be told that they were "unpaid intern jobs". Things went downhill from there. After a few deeply frustrating months applying for jobs and often not even getting a response, let alone an interview, I knew I would have to take matters into my own hands and create my own work. OK, this realisation didn't come that easy. There were lots of tears and many railings at the gods for the world's unfairness.

The first thing I had to do was work out what I wanted to do. I knew I could try freelancing event management or PR and publicity, but I soon realised that what I really wanted to do was to write and get paid for it. I also wanted to see if I could get some radio work.

During my time as PRO for The Alzheimer Society, I had found myself in radio studios on several occasions, and I had always enjoyed it. I love the intimacy of radio. The feeling that you are talking, not to the presenter but to the listener. Just one listener – she could be in her kitchen or driving her car or out for a walk, but she was alone listening to her radio, to you. And I loved that.

But I had never worked in media and knew no one who did. I had no idea how to begin but thought that social media, namely Twitter, might be as good a starting place as any. I had begun to use Twitter in March 2009 by accident – a long story for another book. Back then, it was a quieter, softer place but heavily populated by journalists, editors, presenters, and producers. I set about strategically following anyone I thought could give me an insight into this world about which I knew relatively little. Twitter was also a great place for just chatting and interacting with all manner of people. From those early days, I have made some great friends, people I now know in real life.

A year later, I was following a conversation between some journalists and radio producers about a problem that still dogs media: the lack of women's voices. This online conversation led to a seminar being organised to address the topic and give women interested in going on air some help and tips to do so.

I knew I wanted to be there. I wanted to hear more. So, gathering a small bit of courage in my two hands and prefacing my remarks by saying I was nobody, not a journalist or writer but just interested, I asked if I could attend. There was no problem, and my name was added to the attendee list.

The event was to take place in the National Library in the city on a weekday evening. I didn't want to drive, so I decided to take the bus. I hadn't taken a bus into the city for years. I rarely went into the city anymore. My life was firmly rooted in my suburban locality. Once I figured out the logistics, I realised that I had nothing to wear. I wanted to look a little professional and not like how I felt, which was (and yeah, I know, I hate to admit this now) a housewife who didn't care hugely about how she looked. I dressed for comfort rather than style, of which I had none.

Several times I had thought I would bail out of attending this event, as it all seemed way too complicated. It just seemed like so much hassle. I also needed to make sure someone was home to watch the youngest two. It all felt like a silly indulgence. And of course, I was dogged by the voice in my head that told me I was stupid to think I could ever contribute to media. Who the hell did I think I was?

But something, possibly the need to earn money, kept me onside, and so a few weeks later, I found myself arriving way too early at the National Library for the seminar. As the other attendees began arriving and taking seats, it was clear that the room was almost entirely made up of journalists and other women working in media. And me, the housewife from the burbs. They all knew each other. I knew exactly no one.

But that seminar led to the forming of a committee and a group called Women On Air, and within another year or so, I was on the committee. I had the time that others didn't and knew how to make myself useful.

I began to do a small bit of radio, mainly on news panels. I also started a blog for my writing. A year later, I got my first invitation onto live national TV to do a newspaper review on the Tonight Show on TV3 (now Virgin Media One). It was one of the most terrifying things I have ever done.

The terror one feels when jumping out of your safe place into a new world is real. It is aided and abetted by the voice in your head that keeps telling you that you're an eejit, that you have ideas above your station and that you should go home and make (and eat) more scones. Because you are good at that. And leave the media stuff to the professionals.

But I needed to make some money. I had no choice, and looking back now, I can see that I may not have continued without that impetus. Someone once told me that "fear" is actually just an acronym for "false evidence appearing real". And very often, it is just that. I am not an idiot. I was as entitled to contribute to media as anyone else. However, I can say that and know it's true, but deep in my heart, I am still not convinced – even now, over ten years later.

# THE STORIES

While I was contemplating reinvention and pushing myself out of my comfort zone, I was also becoming aware in a very visceral way that I was ageing. Being in the "over fifties" category can be somewhat sobering. There are exhibitions for the over fifties; there are holidays (usually guided tours or cruises) aimed at the over fifties; there are endless articles and features in magazines about how to dress if you are over 50. All of which is nonsense. (Although to be fair, sometimes there are reductions and special offers for the over-fifties.)

It's just another decade. However, there was an awareness of a clock starting to tick gently in the wings of my life. Its rhythm told me that it was time to get on with stuff. Not bucket-list stuff, no, not yet. But other things that I have always wanted to do. Things like writing a book. Owning a donkey or two, learning to paddleboard. That kind of stuff. It is now time to get on with it.

But just when you feel that added tinge of urgency, you also realise that you no longer have the confidence you may have had when you were younger. The decades before made you wise up to the fact that you are not invincible. You may not even always be right. And your age is beginning to change the way you look. For women, this is a huge issue because we all know that from the time we are little girls, the way we look and present ourselves to the world is hugely important, as it is largely how we are judged. This is not how it should be, but it is.

It is often at around 50 that you catch sight of yourself in a shop window or a mirror, and you wonder who the matronly woman is before realising that it's you. Yes, you have suddenly become your mother.

## Hair Scare

I am a brunette and always have been. I didn't really have an issue with grey hair until I hit 40, and I began to dye my hair. Every few months, I would buy a box of dye with my grocery shopping and lash it in, splattering the far reaches of the bathroom in the process and dyeing towels all shades of brown and russet and auburn. By the time I got to 50, I had realised that the professionals needed to take over my hair colour; they advised me that I might consider going lighter. "Lighter," I said, "I am a brunette. I am not going lighter. But I might go purple." With the benefit of hindsight, I now see that this wanting to go purple was a rage against getting older. I didn't want to be the stereotypical older woman. I wanted the world to know that I was still a bit mad. A bit different. Not that the world cared. But my hairdresser did and refused to dye my hair purple.

So back I went to the supermarket where there was every colour you could imagine, including purple. So, I lashed it in and went purple. Well, it was purple for the first week. Then the top began to go a different shade to the ends, so I had a kind of orangey purple head. But I persevered. I bought more purple. And I went on more holidays, including one to Australia to visit my daughter.

Our usual sloppy, messy reunion was somewhat tempered by her eyes constantly wandering upwards. Finally, she said it: "Jeez Ma, your hair is great craic. It's all kinds of colours." "It's purple," I said. In other words, aren't I the madwoman altogether? When we said goodbye again after two weeks in the heat and the sun and the humidity, her parting words were blunter: "Ma, get your hair sorted. It's shocking and not in a good way."

I finally accepted that my experiment had failed. I called my long-suffering hair salon and begged for an appointment.

As the colourist gently investigated my wondrous hair, she looked me straight in the eye and said, "no-one here did this, did they?" "No", I answered, trying to keep my pride intact, "that's all my own work. But I think maybe I should try to go a bit lighter for the summer."

There: I had said it. Barbara, the life-long brunette, was now officially crossing over to the dark side, well, the blonde side, but you know what I mean.

It wasn't easy. All the red, purple, and orange shades had to be covered first to avoid pink highlights, which I thought sounded interesting. But I shut up and put up. Over the winter, my hair slowly returned to one colour and then got lighter and lighter. So that by that summer, it was blonde.

I tried to tell myself it was for the best. But I didn't feel like me. I kept catching sight of myself and wondering who I was. I tried to like my blonde self. I tried to convince myself that blondes have more fun. But this blonde didn't.

Finally, I cracked. It was back to the hairdressers, who really were patient beyond belief. "I am done with the blonde", I announced. "Bring me back to myself". Two hours later, I was restored. I bounced out of the salon like one of those "I'm worth it" women in the ads. Of course, the joy was short-lived. Within weeks of being re-brunetted, my hair started to return to its natural state. Grey roots on the top of your head are picked up by studio lights and in photos, and I hated them. So, I spent years consulting my diary to see what I had coming up and engaging in all kinds of mental arithmetic as I tried to work out what state my hair would be in on any given date.

This is a fool's game, as it can often mean I left getting my colour done for an extra week because I had an event coming up, and I wanted it to be at its artificial peak for it. And that's always the week when you bump into an old boyfriend or the horrible girl you went to school with and haven't seen in decades. And you know she is thrilled to see you looking so neglected and will gleefully be phoning around her coven to inform them that she bumped into you and you look like shite.

## *Face Ache*

Of course, the other really awful thing that happens as you age is that your face begins to sink and sag. Now let me be straight up about something. I have spent decades putting all manner of chemicals in my hair, but I could never imagine myself having something injected into my face to freeze muscles or plump up my wrinkles. Nope. Getting your hair dyed and blow-dried is a relatively enjoyable experience, but getting injections into my face? Nah. Not for me.

So, my face has softened, like most people my age. In the morning, it looks like a rumpled pillow. Makeup helps, but soft-focus eyesight is better.

Then my passport expired. I was devastated. I loved my passport. With each passing year, I loved it more. As birthdays came and went and I got a year older, my passport photo preserved my face in the year 2008.

With a daughter living overseas and my love of travel and holidays, I have to have an up-to-date passport, so I set about renewing the little burgundy book, which encourages foreign governments to be nice to me and confirms me as a citizen of Ireland. Off to the Garda station for the forms, which I filled out in my best handwriting with my favourite pen. Simple enough. Then for the photo.

Now, this should also be a relatively simple exercise. I am, after all, married to a photographer. Therefore, I don't have to trudge to my nearest shopping centre to sit in a booth clutching a hairbrush and lipstick, then attempt to undo the windblown hair and smudged lips. Oh no, I can have my photo done in the comfort of my own home, standing against the "Summer Solstice" wall in the natural light of the big window, something which my photographer husband assures me is very flattering.

Freshly made up, hair brushed, I was ready.

"Remember you are not allowed to smile anymore," he said. I had forgotten that bit. OK, I decided to do my intelligent look. That's the look I try to adopt when listening to conversations about economics and the stock market. I have always felt it worked quite well.

Click, click, click, click… about twenty images were taken and off I went to inspect the work through the back of the camera.

I was horrified. "Jaysus", I roared at my long-suffering husband, "they're brutal."

I didn't look sad. I looked gutted like a woman who had just learned of some awful tragedy that had befallen her entire family. "I'm not going around the world with a photo like that. Jaysus. Again." And so, he picked up the camera, and I headed back to the Summer Solstice, my mind working overtime.

Maybe I will try enigmatic, I thought. Mysterious. Surely, I could do that without smiling. So, I stood, willing the soft daylight to work its magic and opening my eyes just a little wider than normal in the hope of softening some of my laughter lines. Chins up.

Click, click, click... And back to the camera I went.

"Oh my God." Now I looked not only sad but slightly mad with it. I looked like a woman who had lost her marbles or worse.

I decided I didn't want a bloody passport. I would no longer go abroad. Better for the planet anyway. That seemed better than the ignominy of waving that awful photo in the faces of police forces and immigration officials around the world. We could smile before 9/11. I cursed Osama Bin Laden. Then I wondered why, if my phone can recognise me when I smile, the CIA or FBI or Interpol or whatever can't do likewise? Are we being conned into our awful mugshot passport photos?

I digress. I tried to calm down. The photographer nervously asked if I wanted to try again.

I was out of ideas, except for praying for divine intervention. So, like a prisoner about to be executed, I positioned myself in front of the cream wall again and tried to think positive thoughts.

Click, click, click...

"OK, I now have almost 100 frames. We need to choose one." Which roughly translates as, "I am finished photographing you now, my neurotic wife."

I was close to tears. For the next ten years, I was going to be accompanied on my travels by a photo that reminded me of how gravity and time had conspired to pull my face south, ensuring that when it was "resting", my face wore an expression of huge sadness.

"Maybe if I lay on the bed so that my face went sideways instead of downwards and you stood above me with the camera…"

But the photographer had disappeared, and the door to his office was closed. He was making my print.

In no time at all, we will have to do this again. How sad and mad will I look by then? Just as I was coming to terms with the reality of my face succumbing to the pull of gravity, I hit another disaster.

## *The Break-Up*

One of the real tragedies of getting older and particularly hitting your fifties is that you often find that you cannot drink as you used to anymore. The hangovers become monsters that lurk in the early hours of the morning after, and last and last, sometimes for days. They render you completely useless. Your body objects hugely to your getting drunk, and in the end, for many of us, it takes away all the good things about getting pissed. I still cry when I think about how things used to be.

I had a long and very happy relationship with wine and red wine in particular. We were together longer than I have been married to himself.

I remember well the first bottle of wine I ever bought. Well, I didn't purchase all of it. I had shares in it, so to speak. I was about 14 and walked with a few girl pals over a mile (no – we had shoes, and it wasn't snowing) to a shop where we had heard they weren't very fussed about proof of age when purchasing alcohol. We could afford one bottle between us.

As we neared the shop, it was decided that I alone should enter the premises since I was the tallest, so surely must have looked the oldest. The girls waited around the corner while I completed the transaction without any bother. Then, nursing our precious purchase, we trudged all the way back to the friend's house whose parents were away. Once there, we sat around the kitchen table and, after a long struggle with a corkscrew, managed to get the wine open and carefully doled it out between about five of us.

We were all staying the night, so we went to bed convinced we were all drunk and relishing the thought of hangovers in the morning. Oh, the innocence of it all.

Since those heady schoolgirl days, I have had dalliances with various other tipples. There were the Bacardi & Coke days, the (brace yourself) Malibu & Pineapple days (I feel nauseous just thinking about that, but it was all very *Miami Vice*), and I am still partial to an odd Hot Port or Pear Cider depending on the weather.

But wine... sigh... wine, and I never fell out of love. Oh no, wine has been there every step of the way. From that first bottle of what was most likely Black Tower or Blue Nun to the bottles of Merlot and Shiraz languishing in my wine rack as I type.

I never saw it coming. I thought we were still happily involved in a beautiful relationship, even if it was a relationship that I would admit had its ups and downs. There were some nights (or indeed afternoons) when we overdid our love for each other. There were dawns when I should have been in bed rather than struggling home from a neighbour's house. There were times when the day after the night before was a bit of a struggle because of my overindulgence. However, in fairness, after well over three decades together, we knew each other fairly well, and, like a good marriage, we generally got on pretty well.

In fact, it was better than that. We had some great laughs down the years. The early days of cheap plonk and dodgy corks which disintegrated into the bottle as I struggled to remove them and then had to strain the wine through tights... What? You never did that?

The days spent in Spain drinking rough local vino from earthenware jugs. The cosy, winter nights; me and my wine, together by a roaring fire. All the celebrations, the birthdays, the Christmases... we did them all happily together. Not (necessarily) getting drunk, you understand, but just enjoying each other's company.

But then, as I hit menopause, something changed. At first, I assumed we were just going through a rocky patch.

Two glasses of wine an evening was starting to result in a horrible headache that often woke me in the middle of the night and lasted for most of the following day. As a sufferer of migraines, I tend to get a bit panicky at the onset of a headache. These weren't migraines, but they did leave me feeling pretty awful and very, very tired.

But I persevered, as one does when a relationship has a wobble. I tried to drink water along with the wine. I thought that was helping for a while. But I was only fooling myself.

Then I bought a bottle of white. It's not the same. We just don't have the same chemistry. There were fewer headaches, but there was no spark. No deeply satisfying sigh at the first taste on my lips.

The bottles of red sat looking sadly at me from the rack in the kitchen. So, I decided to risk a glass. Spaghetti bolognese tastes better anyway with a dash of red, so I opened a bottle and poured a glass. I inhaled its spicy aroma deeply. Glass to lips, and that first taste... oh, it was sublime. How I had missed it. But I was sensible – I limited myself to just a glass... and a half.

The next day, I woke at six am with the familiar feeling of my head thumping on the pillow, and my day went slowly south. I cried bitter tears at the realisation that our relationship must end.

Later, I went downstairs and addressed the wine rack. "It's not you", I sobbed, "it's me. I am so sorry, but it's over."

I made do with white wine for a while. Then that started to have the same effect on me. Whole days lost after just a glass. I gave up wine altogether. And I was very sad. So sad that one night I tried to comfort myself with a Bailey's while in the bath, and I lost the next day to a migraine. So, I made a momentous decision. I had to give up alcohol. It was all over. Menopause is great craic altogether.

Like a jilted lover, I lived in the hope that we may be reunited one day, so I never disposed of my haul of red wine bottles that carry on winking and whistling at me every time I walk past. I like the fact that they were still close by. But I do have regrets. Jokes really are much funnier when you're drunk. Colours are brighter. And you have more energy, especially at one or two in the morning. It was hard not drinking. Because in Ireland, unless you are pregnant or on antibiotics, giving up alcohol makes you, well, weird. And not in a cool way.

I managed over two years completely off the drink. It was a pain in the ass. And every so often, I would experiment with a glass of wine (white, not red) to see if I could get away with it. I generally couldn't.

Menopause symptoms began to abate somewhat, so one day I tried gin. Just one gin and tonic. And no headache. It was the start of my return into the arms of the odd drink. I am pleased to tell you that I can now enjoy ONE G&T or ONE glass of wine. Yes, it does help me to feel special again, but I still miss that warm, fuzzy feeling you get as you slide deliciously down into the warm bath of inebriation. Because surely that's the point of alcohol, isn't it? Drinking in moderation is fine and good when you are trying not to make a fool of yourself... But sometimes, you desperately want to make a fool of yourself. You desperately want the world to seem like a giant cartoon. You want to cry with laughter at stupid stuff that you can only do when pissed. The wild abandonment that comes with being well soaked in gin or wine or whatever. God, but I still miss it.

## Feminism

I always knew I was a feminist. Growing up in such a male household made me realise early that I would have to stand up for myself and demand what I thought was my fair dues. However, it probably took me until my fifties to be happy being labelled a feminist – yeah, I know, I know. I am mortified to admit that. And no, I don't know why I wasn't comfortable with the title. But in my fifties, I gave it lots of thought and realised it was past time to nail my colours to the mast and give an example to my girls by taking my feminism out of the closet and wearing it with pride.

On one of my first forays onto daytime TV on the *Midday* show (latterly called *Elaine*) on TV3 (now Virgin Media), we discussed feminism and equality. And I stupidly said something like, "but what is feminism exactly, how to you define it?" And a much younger, brighter panellist said, "of course you can define feminism; it's in the dictionary, Barbara," or words to that effect. I was mortified. But I learned a valuable lesson that day. Well, two lessons. Always be prepared when contributing to a debate. And, more importantly, especially as you get older, review your opinions regularly.

That day in the television studio, I wasn't sure if I wanted to be called a feminist. I thought it sounded too aggressive. I know, I know. I had somehow absorbed a lot of the negativity that the patriarchy put out about women demanding equality, and that was coupled with my subconscious need to be liked, something I think a lot of women and girls suffer from. After making a tit of myself on live TV, I went home and read a lot about feminism and got brave; although I know, now it's not really bravery. I realised that, of course, I am a feminist. I have always been a feminist. Of course. I believe that women should be treated equally to men and have equal opportunities. And if my calling myself a feminist is a problem for some people, it ain't *my* problem.

However, being a feminist can often be a right pain in the ass. It makes life more complicated and difficult. It can screw stuff up and make your head explode. In fact, at times, it can be downright depressing. It can feel so much easier not to see the inequality and accept the status quo.

I sometimes envy the old me, who didn't think too deeply about many things and found it easier to ignore stuff that I thought I was unlikely to be able to fix.

Emer O'Toole, the feminist academic and columnist, described the three stages of feminism as initially having the "scales patriarchy so painstakingly glued to your eyeballs fall away". She describes the second stage as "a searingly painful period during which all you can see is gender inequality and sexism, where once there was a meritocracy and cheeky banter. You feel powerless. You can't shut up about it. No one invites you to dinner parties." She describes the third stage as when you start seeking out other feminists to change the world.

I must be a slow learner because I seem to be eternally stuck in the second stage, and it is painful. It is excruciating to suddenly see sexism where you were previously blissfully ignorant. It can make the most innocent of pursuits seem fraught with danger. Sometimes I think how simpler life would be if I wasn't a feminist.

I first thought this was some years ago when I was driving back from West Cork to Dublin. Music is the key to good motorway driving, but the music must be familiar, so you can sing along. I had recently discovered how to connect Spotify on my phone to the car's stereo, so I announced to my music-mad daughter (who was about 15 at the time) that I was going to share with her some of my favourite songs from my formative years. The great music of the 1970s.

Some of this she was familiar with, as she a big fan of Queen. So, we began by singing (well, she sings, I kind of roar) "You're My Best Friend" and "Somebody to Love". Then my playlist shuffled along and threw up Rod Stewart's "Tonight's the Night". Daughter was unfamiliar and so stayed quiet, while I found myself roaring ", come on Angel, my heart's on fire. Don't deny your man's desire," and if you know the song, you will know that the following two lines are even worse. My brain did a flip as I made a mental note to jettison that particular ditty from my playlist. In fairness, it was never one of his best.

Some good Motown followed, and I bellowed along happily to Aretha and Gloria. Then Dr Hook started warbling, "when your body has had enough of me, and I'm laying out on the floor, and when you think I've loved you all that I can, I'm gonna love you a little more."

I decided to get daughter to change the playlist from the 70s and suggested some Neil Diamond, as my mother was also in the car, and he is one of her favourites. It has to be said that I am partial to a bit of Mr Diamond too. First up – yep, you've guessed it, "girl, you'll be a woman soon, and soon you'll need a man."

All this misogynistic awfulness was thrown into stark relief by the fact that, before I left Bantry (West Cork), I had spent two hours in a room full of feminists who had gathered to listen to feminist writer and icon, Gloria Steinem.

My head was starting to hurt. And ashamed as I am to admit it, I fudged the issue with my daughter. Instead of having a conversation about sexual consent, I mumbled something about how you wouldn't get away with those lyrics today. And as I did, I could hear the collective sigh of the sisterhood as they despaired at my letting them all down.

A year or two later, I found myself in the car with all my daughters, who were then aged 30, 19 and 17, along with my baby granddaughter, on our way home after some Christmas shopping when I casually remarked that I was looking forward to Christmas. My utterance triggered the following exchange:

Eldest: "Really? I am surprised you said that without adding something about all the so-called 'crass commercialism.'"

Me: "Well yeah, there is that. But it's still nice to have a mid-winter celebration."

Middle: "Seriously? I am surprised you haven't embarked on a rant about how Santa is a man, and why isn't he a woman. Imagine Ma. Why isn't Santa Claus, Sandra Claus?"

Me: "What?"

Eldest: "Yeah, and speaking of Mrs Claus – what kind of a woman is she anyway, in the kitchen baking and all that. And she didn't even keep her own name. She doesn't even have a first name. Some feminist she is."

Me: "Em…"

Youngest: "True, and all the reindeer are male too. Not a doe among them. Not one. Does that not bother you, Ma? Not very gender balanced, is it?"

The joy I had been feeling was sucked out of the car as I pondered if, in fact, I am the

feminist who stole Christmas… from my children? Well, adult children. But still.

Of course, it's all advertisers' fault, really. The Coca Cola company is generally responsible for the jolly red-suited man we love today. Mrs Claus, however, has traditionally been a shadowy figure, usually depicted as an elderly, white-haired woman in a fur-trimmed outfit who spends most of her time in the kitchen or overseeing the elves.

That particular year Marks and Spencer tried to reimagine her as a kind of female James Bond who delivered special toys by snowmobile and helicopter. Except being "the good woman" she was, she kept her endeavours secret, letting the big man take all the kudos. I found this very disappointing. Old Mrs Claus in the kitchen was a more convincing feminist than Bond Claus. It takes more than a power suit and sassy attitude, don't you know?

But the lack of gender balance in the reindeer is a real problem. What is that about? Are we to believe that girl reindeer are worse drivers than boy reindeer? Or would having a few girls in the team cause them to get lost? Or perhaps the entire endeavour on

Christmas Eve night would run late? Like, seriously? We need some does in there, amongst

Rudolph and Donner and Blitzen et al. I mean, think of the children, at least the baby girl reindeer. How can a young doe be what she cannot see?

However, all is not as it seems. Some cursory research points to the fact that, although none seem to have female names, it is most likely that Santa's reindeer ARE, in fact, female. Rudolph and his mates are usually depicted with antlers and sisters, it's the female reindeer that hold onto their antlers, while the male reindeer shed theirs in winter.

Added to that is the fact that female reindeer also retain more fat, making them better able to cope with the long journey around the world in the cold mid-winter. The concept of flying reindeer originates in old Northern European pagan folk tales about a great Goddess who took to the sky on the darkest night, the Winter Solstice, to bring back the light, and she was pulled by her reindeer. Christianity or the patriarchy or something wasn't having any of that, of course, and so, well, you know the rest. The female reindeer went the way that women in history often do, airbrushed out of the story altogether. Think of the women of 1916 Rising, the women in NASA in the early days of space flight, and countless other women lost in HIStory.

So, Mrs Claus is the real power in the Claus household, although she gets little credit, something many women who work in the home I am sure can identify with. And Santa's reindeer with their male names are most likely Does, female deer.

OK, so this is tongue in cheek, but both these examples serve to illuminate the fact that feminism makes life complicated. But it's vital if women are to change the world – and boy, do we need to change the world. We must begin by seeing all the inequality that is often right under our noses, although somehow, we can remain blind to it.

There are still too many conference panels where there are NO WOMEN or just the token female among a sea of men. There are still TV panel shows where there is one female in a panel of four or more. Radio in Ireland has certainly improved in the last ten years, but women are still in the minority of the voices we hear. There is a particular problem in local radio, which hasn't made the progress the nationals have. As I write, there is a campaign underway to ensure that female musicians are more equally represented on music radio. And it is up to all of us who believe in equality to call this out. But be aware – it won't make you popular.

I have been at awards dinners where I have made myself a bit of a pariah by asking why so few women were receiving awards or why there are so few women working in the particular industry represented. But it is vital that we all do this to make this world a better place for our daughters and granddaughters. It is up to us to shine our light on instances of low or no representation of women and to keep asking why. Because in my experience, it is often just the accepted norm, and no one has thought to wonder why yet.

## THE WISDOM TAKEAWAYS

I was in my forties, busy with young kids, when I realised that I had turned into my mother, as I regularly found myself uttering the exact words she had used on me when I was a child. You know what I am talking about...

"Because I said so."

"This is not a restaurant, there is no choice on the menu."

"Shut the bloody door – were you born in a barn?"

And no, I still don't really know what that means either. Didn't stop me from using it, though.

But it was in my fifties when I realised that I now not only sounded like her, but I was beginning to look like her too. Many days, especially when I am tired or just out of bed, I am confronted with my image in the mirror, and I see my mother staring back at me. It is a sobering experience that sums up what your fifties can be about.

During this decade, women must make peace with getting older and the physical changes that brings with it.

I am not just talking about menopause but the changes to your hair, figure, and skin. You need to decide around now whether you are going to embark on a potentially expensive, time-consuming project to "fight ageing" (of which more anon), or you make peace with the fact you are getting older and accept it so that you can move on and make the most of these years. That doesn't mean giving up on how you look but having realistic expectations. Don't beat yourself up for looking – well… middle-aged. This is the decade when women should refuse to be defined by how we look. Equally, we need to work hard on no longer caring about what others think about how we look.

My fifties have been another decade of ups and downs, highs and lows. It has been a decade where I did that thing that many women who have spent years running a home and looking after kids do: wondering, "who am I?" I am that mama bird whose chicks still live in the nest but are fully-fledged every way but financially and no longer need me to be there for them all the time.

This can be difficult for women, especially in a society that places no value on the work involved in caring (be it for children, elderly parents or vulnerable adults) or running a home. Our society only values that which creates monetary wealth, so our work is seen as something that should be done in the margins of life. So, when that period of life is coming to an end, I think many women find themselves wondering what to do next. And this holds true whether you have been at home with your kids or are busy in the corporate world, where retirement may be coming over the horizon.

As I attempted to reinvent myself, I learned a very important thing that surprised me, much to my own shame. It is that women are in general very supportive of other women. My journey from my suburban kitchen to being a media contributor was only made possible by a legion of women (and indeed some great men, too) who have supported me. In fact, they not only supported me, but they cheered me on. They had made themselves available to me when I needed to ask stupid questions. They never made me feel the eejit that the voice in my head still regularly tells me I am. And many of these women are radio producers who took a chance on me and put me on air when I had very few air miles in the bank.

We regularly hear how bitchy women are to each other, especially in workplaces. In my experience, this is simply nonsense. The writers and journalists who have given me the confidence to do my thing have been anything but bitchy. They have been wonderful supporters.

I have learnt to take a risk and to trust myself. I have learnt that making a mistake or failing at something (and believe me, I have done both, and sometimes spectacularly) only makes you like everyone else. Everyone successful has made mistakes. It's part and parcel of how we learn and grow. I now realise that being at home for a decade doing a job that society places no value on means that I still have a way to go when it comes to believing in my own abilities. So, I'm still working on my confidence.

However, I have almost learned to tell the voice in my head to shut the fuck up. And I have realised that it really is as easy as that – simply telling it to shut the fuck up. I have learned that I am not my mind. My mind, just like my arm or my leg, can be controlled by my brain. My mind often serves up nonsense. So does yours.

Most of all, I have realised that I am about to embark on what could potentially be one of the most productive, fulfilling decades of my life. I have the experience, the freedom, and thankfully, the energy to make some of my long-held dreams – big and small – happen. Bring it on.

# LOOK BACK AT YOUR FIFTIES

**It's a big birthday** – So, how did it feel to turn 50? Were you depressed about it, happy enough or neither?

**Making peace with getting older** – If you are in your fifties or older, have you made peace with getting older and all the changes that brings to how we look. Are you engaged in "fighting ageing", and how do you feel about that? Which worries you more, your health or your appearance?

**Identity crisis** – This is often the decade when retirement from the workplace is in the middle distance, and the kids are more or less fully-fledged, so how does that feel?

Have you got an empty nest? Are you wondering who this "you" is now that you can perhaps contemplate life without having to work so hard and without having to actively care for children?

**Feminism** – Have you thought about feminism at this stage in your life? Have you wondered about how life has been thus far for you as a woman? How do you feel about that?

**Expectations vs reality** – as you began your fifties, what were your expectations and how have they panned out?

# I AM WOMAN, HEAR ME ROAR

Helen Reddy's lyrics will most likely be familiar to most women of my age. Back in 1972, in a song that helped define the women's movement in America, she sang:

*"I am woman, hear me roar*

*In numbers too big to ignore*

*And I know too much to go back and pretend*

*'Cause I've heard it all before*

*And I've been down there on the floor*

*No one's ever gonna keep me down again*

*Oh yes I am wise*

*But it's wisdom born of pain*

*Yes, I've paid the price*

*But look how much I gained*

*If I have to, I can do anything*

*I am strong*

*I am invincible*

*I am woman"*

So, as we move forward into our freedom years, listen to Helen's words of wisdom, and listen to them regularly. Because she nailed it. You are strong. You are invincible. You are woman.

Now is the time to gather that quilt of memories, stories, and experiences around you and start to dream about this new phase of life. Start to visualise how you would like to spend the coming years. Now is the time to mind your health so that you will have the energy to make the most of these delicious years ahead. You are creating your legacy.

However, more than that, you are making a difference. You are redefining what it is to be an older woman by sharing your experiences and your stories. And redefining older women's place in our world for not just our daughters and granddaughters but for our sons too.

# COULD OUR SIXTIES BE THE BEST DECADE YET?

*"A heart without a dream is like a bird without feathers."*

**Suzi Kassem**

For the last four chapters, I have used the decades of my own life to look back at some of the defining elements of each period. I began the last chapter by expressing how I expected the meaning of life to be revealed to me when I turned 50. However, disappointingly, there was no flash of inspiration or insight as to what it was all about. In most ways, I feel no wiser than I was at 20. However, looking back and cumulatively assessing my life so far, I realise that I have the tools, the experience, and the stories at my disposal now, which just might help make this next decade the most powerful yet.

My fifties have been a time of transformation as I gave up various roles that I had actively played for decades and sought my own renaissance as a writer and broadcaster. I have passed through the portal of menopause and am just beginning to sense the beauty, the peace, the calm, and the power of the space I am about to enter. This space, along with my accumulated experience, makes me so excited for this next decade… my sixties.

There has never been a better time to be getting older than right now. For women, it can be a tricky age to navigate, although it shouldn't be because getting older can be a wonderful liberation. Once we have negotiated the tricky waters of menopause, we should be able to cruise gloriously into a very powerful time of our life. Some women don't get to experience any or all of their sixties. By the time you have arrived here, you will likely have lost a friend or two to cancer or heart disease or some other health issue. Even those of us who get to 60 in reasonable nick, many of us feel that we are fading away slowly as we experience a crisis of confidence and have difficulty working out exactly who we are now.

Post-menopausal women are like salmon, swimming upstream against the tide, knowing deep in our bones that we have a dream to hatch. But we are constantly thwarted by the bullshit that all women are fed, particularly women over 50. We live in a society that places no value on ageing, especially if you are a woman. This means it can be difficult to make peace with our ageing as we are diverted into all kinds of self-sabotaging behaviour and thus miss the opportunity to step into our power, to become the dynamic older woman that is our birthright. This is not only a huge disappointment for us individually but an enormous loss for society and for our planet as a whole.

I firmly believe that, once we have weathered all the weird shit that menopause can throw at us – some expected (hot flashes, mood swings) and some not so much (hay fever, who knew?) – women can move into what can and should be the most satisfying phase of our lives. And there is nothing to mark that. There is nothing to celebrate that, as a woman gets older, she should naturally be moving into her full power and truest self. There is so much to celebrate about post-menopausal life.

# DELICIOUS FREEDOM

By the age of 50, most women are on the verge of menopause if not already fully engaged with all the joys it brings; itchy skin, periods that come out of nowhere, aching joints, etc. But hey, at least we are unlikely to become pregnant. In this decade, most of us will have finally arrived in a place where our baby-making biology will have receded completely for the first time since we were girls.

For nigh on 40 years, women will have coped with school, exams, college, more exams, work, travel, relationships, and children, while also coping with the monthly mess which causes logistical problems that men never even have to fully comprehend, let alone have to deal with.

With apologies to Dr King, it is post-menopause when we will arrive at a time when we are "free at last, free at last, thank God almighty..." As women of a certain age know, you are deemed to be officially in menopause when a year has passed without you menstruating. Well, why the hell aren't we throwing parties? Freedom from bleeding and all the accompanying side effects means that we are also (more or less – be careful) finally free of our fertility.

Fertility is a precious gift and one that most women experience with joy. However, being the ones who get pregnant means that we will forever be the ones who worry most about getting pregnant. We have spent decades trying desperately to get pregnant or trying desperately not to get pregnant. So, menopause delivers no more worries in this respect. From now on, there are no more contraceptive pills, diaphragms, coils or other medieval-sounding devices to ensure those sneaky sperm don't get to our baby eggs. Sure, that right there is enough of a reason to be delighted you are now in your fifties. And OK, I know all about vaginal dryness... but I am a glass half full woman about this. There's always lube.

## Space in your Head

OK, so once you become a mother, you will always be a mother... and your kids, big adults though they might be, will still be in occasional need of your wisdom, cups of tea, your fabulous lasagne, and a hug that only a mammy can give. I know that. However, your kids are most likely more or less independent by this time. They may not have moved out, but your days of active parenting are over.

Your time is finally your own. You have spent years and years making packed lunches, going to parent-teacher meetings, doing school runs, minding sick kids, and taking them to doctors/dentists/orthodontist appointments. In fact, for years, you probably put their needs ahead of yours. Now, you can finally come and go as you please. The sweet, sweet freedom that you probably dreamed of for years is finally here. Too often, instead of grabbing this freedom with both hands, women remain stuck actively cooking, washing, and cleaning for adult children who really are capable of looking after themselves.

Now, I am not saying that if you are home and cooking dinner you should just make your own once your kids are adults. Of course not. What I am saying is that you have a choice. Take off that apron and grab opportunities that were impossible for you until now. As they become adults, your kids must know that you are ALSO seeking more independence. So, if there is a class, a concert, or whatever you would like to go to, go. And don't feel that you must leave dinner in the microwave. Just go. Not only will they be fine, but it's good for them to realise that (a) they can manage and (b) you have a life too.

As a mother, you have had a large part of your brain dedicated to "kids' stuff" for decades. You held all their individual preferences there, what food they liked and what they didn't. What books they had read, their favourite movies, what cartoons they liked, who their friends were, what those friends' moms' names were, and where they lived. You also remembered vaccinations, dental check-ups and doctors' appointments. You knew their teachers' names, kept track of homework and supervised it when they were little. You knew what extra-curricular activities they had on what day and arranged complicated rotas with other parents to get them there and back. You always kept spare birthday cards and even presents for last-minute birthday party invitations – in other words, the invites you find when they are a week old and smeared with butter or yoghurt at the bottom of their school bag.

As they got older, you helped with subject choices, kept them as calm as possible before exams and, once they got underway, made sure you cooked their favourite dinners every evening. You picked up the pieces when their hearts got broken for the first time. You saw then through the nonsense of such modern rites of passage such as 6th Year holidays and the Debs. You collected them, delivered them, and waited in the city for their safe arrival out of the "junior disco". You did it all.

Whether you worked outside the home or not, you can now retrieve that bit of yourself that belonged to your kids. Because it's now OVER. Well, it's more or less over!

Your head is finally your own, except for the bit they still inhabit, which causes you to worry about them. According to my 86-year-old ma, that bit remains forever. In general, though, you have got extra brain space: space you can use to figure out what it is you want. Space where you can begin to plant the seeds of reinvention. Space to think about how you might want the next phase of your life to develop. This space is for your dreams, of which more anon.

## *Other People's Opinions; So What?*

Most of us begin to notice a subtle change in our attitude to what people think of us at around 40. By 50, there is a very definite sense of giving far less fucks as to what others really think of you or how you choose to live your life. By the age of 60, if you haven't found this particular freedom yet – listen up and then make an effort. It's the greatest gift. The fear of being judged is one of the biggest barriers to change. You need to dump those fucks.

I am not suggesting for one minute that we get to the point where we become completely selfish, pursuing our own agenda regardless of how it may affect others, especially those we love. But for centuries, girls have been brought up to be people-pleasers, nice, polite, and gentle; these lessons, which are learned early, often get further cemented into place as we get older.

At home, we learn to put our own needs last. We care for our children, ageing parents, and partners and run our homes. OK, so every now and then, we may have a blowout when the pressure mounts, but in general, women grin and bear the fact that we are still doing the lion's share of the housework and caring. All the research says that no matter how many of you might have a "new man" who actually does his fair share, he's still in the minority. Women still do all the heavy lifting in running a home and caring.

In the workplace, if we become assertive, we are often labelled "shrill" or "cranky" or "'bossy" or "irrational" –there is no shortage of terms that are reserved purely to describe women who are a bit "strident" (yep, another one). Some of us relish being troublesome and couldn't care less what names we are called. However, for most women trying to juggle it all, being perceived as "nice" just makes life easier.

Well, let me tell you, sisters, once you get past menopause, those days are over. You realise you aren't bothered anymore about what people think about you. You realise that what other people think about you is their business, not yours. I am not sure why this change in our attitudes happens. Perhaps it's just that we get too tired to bother. Perhaps we realise just how precious our mental health is and that worrying about what others think about you is a sure way to wreck your head. Whatever the reason, when I turned 40 and with every decade since I have less and less fucks to give. It's liberating, I tell you.

There was a magnificent tweet by @janee, a woman on a mission to make 50+ women "uninvisible". She tweeted on 27th February 2019:

*"Just found an unexpected upside to being 55+ start-up founder. Been so busy readying for the launch of #uninvisibility that I've fallen behind on household tasks. Ran out of knickers days ago. Who knew going commando was so easy post-menopause? #startupstress #sayourage*

This says it all really... beautifully illustrating the freedom from biology and all the logistics of periods along with the freedom of not caring what anyone thinks.

## SO... WHAT DO YOU WANT?

"So, tell me what you want, what you really, really want...," sang five young women from the UK back in 1996. OK, they were singing to our daughters, but we heard the song too, and the question, like the song, is lodged in our brains. This question becomes even more valid as we cruise into our post-menopausal stage of life and find ourselves wondering what's next. What do we want; what do we really, really want? How are we going to make the most of this time? Could our sixties be the defining decade of our lives?

I am not entirely sure what I want, and if you aren't either, perhaps we need to ask ourselves what we dream of. What do we fantasise about (easy, easy)?

I sometimes catch a glimpse of another life, a life that is just beyond the periphery of my imagination. I am currently trying to catch these dreams, these visions, some of which are only misty notions that inhabit my nighttime, because I know that right now, I am on the cusp of being able to make these dreams a reality. I urge you to begin doing the same and remember they needn't be huge life-changing dreams. They can be as simple as taking up pottery, painting, or re-joining the paid workforce. Although that last one can be tricky when you are a woman in her sixth decade. Ageism and sexism collide beautifully in capitalism.

Even if you manage to make your dreams clear, women are so used to taking into account the repercussions of our actions on other people that we often tend to park those dreams until some unspecified time in the future. By the time you reach 60, though, you know there is a finite window between the freedom of these years and the day when you might not have the energy or physical ability to pursue them. The time to make these dreams happen may never be perfect... but this time, right now, may be the closest you will come to it being possible.

# DREAM STORIES

## *The superpower of being brought up Catholic*

Like most Irish people my age, I had a very Catholic upbringing. My family went to Mass every Sunday. I clearly remember putting my foot down when I was about 14 and declaring that I didn't need to go every week. It seemed like such a rebellion at the time, but after some mild opposition, my parents agreed to it. More astounding is the fact that I also went to confession every Saturday of my own volition for much of my childhood. There was a period between the ages of about eight to eleven when my Saturday mornings consisted of confession followed by an hour at drama class. Drama class was a real treat that I looked forward to all week, but apparently, confession was an absolute necessity.

Looking back, it seems so ridiculous that it's funny; shuffling into a pitch-black box to gaze into a priest's ear while I "confessed" to the same sins, most of which I hadn't actually committed because in the back of my mind was the vague threat of something awful happening if I didn't go through this weird ritual every week. In keeping with the monotony of my sins, I always got the same penance, three 'Hail Marys', which I quickly murmured in the church before racing on to my drama class. We were such sheep, including our parents. We questioned every little and accepted all kinds of madness;

177

as we now know, this passivity kept much cruelty and abuse hidden.

I was the child who took part in Corpus Christi processions; on Good Friday, I even went with my friends to do the Stations of the Cross, which I must admit I hated. I hate stories that contain torture, violence, and horror. I have always hated crucifixes. I would burn every single one in a big bonfire if I could, especially the ones that were once (perhaps they still are) all over our hospitals. What an image to gaze upon as you try to recover your health.

I digress again. My school days, and indeed my children's, were liberally soaked in Catholicism. I went to a national school (and Irish national schools are still largely an arm of the church), and, in secondary school, I was educated by the nuns. (It has to be said that this was mainly a positive experience for me.)

All this religion, Catholicism, in particular, gave me a gift for using my imagination. To be part of most religions, you must have a rich inner life; in other words, you must suspend your disbelief to imagine all the mad stuff. Come on, you know what I mean. The old man God, the father. The slightly trendier Jesus, who I do still have time for. In addition, the much sidelined Mary, who got pregnant without even having sex and is supposedly the mother of God. It's gas how she was an actual single mother, but Mary Magdalene, the supposedly "fallen woman" (prostitute in other words), is the icon that the church decided was the appropriate patron saint of fallen Irish women. Women who actually did have sex and, like Mary, got pregnant outside of "wedlock" (although admittedly not with the son of God) were incarcerated into Magdalene Laundries to provide slave labour for the religious orders that ran them. These institutions also served as a punishment for these women's wicked ways while keeping them hidden from view lest their immoral deeds infect the rest of society.

Where was I? Oh yes, imagination. Being a good Catholic girl, I used my imagination when I was young. It has been one of the most useful gifts the Catholic Church bestowed on me, one in which I have found refuge throughout my life.

(I should also say at this point that I have since relinquished my membership of the Catholic Church.)

Of course, nowadays, this ability to entertain all kinds of stuff in your mind is referred to as visualisation, the art of imagining something you wish to connect with or achieve in great detail. In addition to my dreaming skills, as a child, I was also a voracious reader, which further harnessed the power of my imagination.

I ate up everything Enid Blyton wrote. From the Four Marys through to Mallory Towers and from the Famous Five to the Secret Seven, her books were hugely important to me as a child. Books provide a perfect escape from the world we inhabit in a way that TV doesn't. You can half-watch a TV programme, but you cannot half-read a book. You must pay attention to what you are reading, and a book can spirit you away to all kinds of other worlds, albeit in my case, very British "jolly hockey sticks" worlds that were light years away from the one I inhabited.

I also read poetry. I was extremely lucky to have had the most wonderful teacher right through my primary school years. A teacher who loved words, who I credit with my own love of the written word. She made us listen to poetry well above our pay grade in junior school. She used to say that it wasn't so that we could understand it but just so that we could appreciate the beauty of the language and the imagery. She read us poetry in Irish so that we could listen to the lyricism of our native tongue. She was a wonderful teacher doing what all good teachers do. She didn't just teach; she opened our young minds to all kinds of possibilities.

She also encouraged us in our "creative writing" – essays and poetry. My poetry prowess didn't reach its zenith until I was a teenager, when I poured all my angst, both general and specific, onto the pages of a notebook I kept specifically for this purpose.

Daydreaming? So what, I hear you say. Daydreaming provides us with a way to comfort, distract and soothe ourselves and instil hope into our lives. It is a much-underrated activity. As far as I am concerned, its main purpose is to help us understand what it is that we really want.

Daydreaming is free and available almost anytime to anyone. I daydream in the bath and in the car, where I also sometimes talk to myself about my daydreams. Nowadays, people assume you are on the phone, but I have been talking to myself in the car for decades. I also daydream while hanging out washing, walking the dog and before I go to sleep and do some real dreaming.

## Dreams Of A Place Of My Own

I guess the first time I recognised the latent superpower of dreaming was when I was about 25. As you know, I was one of those fallen women with a baby and without the decency to have a boyfriend, never mind an actual husband. I was finding life quite challenging. I had a toddler and was living at home with my family, who were extremely supportive. However, it was a busy house. There were my three brothers, my uncle with the learning disability, Ma and Da, and myself and baby – eight of us – with one bathroom. It was almost a tenement. (Relax – I know it wasn't, I am being facetious.)

Let me be clear – attempting to parent for the first time, alone and under the gaze of three brothers, all of whom were younger than me, and quite entertained that their seemingly sensible older sister had managed to fall quite spectacularly from her pedestal, wasn't easy.

Sharing a room with a toddler wasn't ideal either, so I spent hours dreaming of another life. These daydreams didn't include a Prince Charming charging in on a white horse to rescue me and bring me to a suburban semi-detached with a garden and a sunny kitchen. My dreams were far more modest but were strongly focused on finding my own place. A place to call home. My home. For my daughter and me. It is a place where we would be safe, warm, and comfortable, something you take for granted until you don't have it.

At this time, my friend Rita (she of the champagne) and her husband had moved to live in rural Wicklow, where they built their own spacious house. I would regularly head south to spend a night or two with them as a form of respite. This option saved my sanity on several occasions. I am not sure if they ever realised just how much I needed those nights in their home.

However, the point is that my journey up and down to Wicklow took me past a building that used to fascinate me. It was so modest that I thought maybe, just maybe, I could afford to rent it. It was up a narrow lane, just visible from the main road and looked as if it might have been a small shop in a previous life. Above the shop front and accessed by external stone stairs was what looked like a small flat. Probably two rooms and a bathroom. I didn't think beyond the fact that it might possibly be affordable. The fact that my daughter's crèche was miles away, as was my work, didn't enter my daydream because I just wanted somewhere that I could call my own. Somewhere I could close the door, and it would be just my daughter and me.

That dream sustained me for a while until I became more ambitious. Small townhouses developments started to spring up around Dublin suburbs in the '90s. There was one in particular that I daydreamed about all the time.

It was just up the road from our family home and opposite the school, I had gone to. This development of about 20 neat and tidy looking townhouses was set around a green space. Perfect for a mammy with a small girl to look after. And it was very close to my own mammy. I think what really made me dream of living there was that these houses were built on the site of an old dairy. A place of which I had been extremely fond.

Suttons TEK Dairy had been an institution in the area when I was a child. Sutton was the family's name who owned the dairy, which they named after a famous battle at Tel El Kebir in Egypt in which some Irish battalions of the British Army were involved. It was an exotic name, which suited the magical place where a hooter rang out three times a day announcing the start of the workday, lunchtime and going-home time. The open yard gave a view into the inner workings of the bottling and the carousel from which the milk bottles hung by their necks, swinging around and around all day. The best thing about the dairy was the horses. The huge, dray horses pulled the milk carts around suburban south county Dublin right into the '70s. I can still hear them as they clip-clopped down our road and stopped every few houses to give the milkman a chance to drop the bottles on the relevant doorsteps and collect the empties.

My school days were punctuated by that hooter; there was also a dairy shop to buy sweets after school. I was convinced that all these echoes were still captured within the green courtyard where the new townhouses had been built. All signs of the dairy were long gone, although the name Tel El Kebir survives to this day in a local football club – TEK United.

I went to view the show house when they first went on the market, even though I had no savings for a deposit, let alone enough income to pay a mortgage. But I knew in my bones that dreaming was keeping me sane.

I spent years dreaming about how I would like every room in my house to look and feel. I grew up in a house that had a lot of magnolia walls, and perhaps that's why I love the colours of the Caribbean or India. Perhaps it's the Irish climate, which delivers so much rain and grey skies, draining the landscape of colour, that makes me crave vibrant interiors.

Along with lots of colours, I dreamed of a country kitchen with a Belfast sink and a range, squishy sofas, and most of all, an open fire. The open fire is one of those increasingly rare things that connects my childhood to my mother's but which is also a thread that stretches back through the generations of our ancestors who gathered around a fire to talk, dream, and cook. There is something primitive about a fire. The magic of an open fire with the crackle of wood and the flickering light softens everything, from faces to voices and minds. And, of course, a fireside is an ideal place to dream.

My daydream bedroom was very much at odds with my otherwise traditional vibe because, when I tried to visualise it, I generally saw a Bedouin tent, resplendent lanterns, huge cushions, throws and, again, the hot colours that for me are the epitome of comfort.

So, I hear you think, was your first home just like your dreams? No, clearly it wasn't. But that's not the point. The point is that those dreams of a home of my own, detailed dreams in which I visualised every room in some detail, were what kept me sane. Years and years later, when himself and I bought our first home, I had some idea of how I would want it to look, but more importantly, how I wanted it to feel.

# NEW LIFE IN A NEW PLACE

As I contemplate my sixties, the idea of a different life, just out of my field of vision, is a constant daydream. I am increasingly aware that there may be another Barbara waiting to be born: another version of myself that is currently starting to wriggle against the cocoon of my life. A me who is dying to take the freedom that is tantalisingly close at hand now. The anchor – well, there are two of them – to my current life are my two college student kids. But freedom is coming, so all this exploration of alternative lives in my head is useful research.

So, where might this new life take place? I doubt that I could ever leave Ireland permanently. However, there may be an opportunity to rent our house in the coming years and take a year out in another country. We might be able to sample life under the sun, even if only for a couple of months. And I know the places I might head to. There are a few options.

## *Puerto De La Cruz*

I have long been a Hispanophile. My love of Spain began when I became captivated by some tiny black and white photos in an old biscuit tin at home.

My mother spent a year in Seville in the 1950s when she was 19, teaching English in a convent school in a village outside the Andalusian capital. She was there for Feria (the April Fair), and although the photos were in black and white, the colour and excitement were palpable, especially to a ten-year-old growing up in 1970s Ireland. It all looked so exotic. To add to the exoticism, Ma also fell in love with a chap called Rafael, who was a bit short to be called dashing but was certainly very cute. So, from an early age Spain, with all its colourful glamour, appealed to me.

I first visited when I was 13, and we took our first family package holiday abroad. Some six or seven years later, I first visited a place that has retained a special place in my heart. That place is the island of Tenerife, the largest of the Canary Islands – more specifically, the town of Puerto de la Cruz in the north. I first visited when I was working in the travel business and went to the island with a colleague on a familiarisation trip.

We had spent two nights in the busy resorts in the south of the island and then made our own way north to visit Puerto de la Cruz – the original tourist destination in Tenerife. Although still thriving in the '80s, it had begun to decline towards the end of the century as holidaymakers favoured the newer resorts in the south. We were to take the local bus north and had been warned to get the bus marked "Directo" because otherwise, we would end up on the slow bus, which went up over the mountains. Needless to say, we got on the wrong bus, which instead of heading out and onto the motorway towards Santa Cruz, took what looked like a Canarian boreen which headed uphill, snaking its way north.

We settled down for what was clearly going to be a long journey. However, only a mile or two later, the bus pulled into a tiny, dusty village and came to a halt. The male passengers disembarked along with the bus driver. The women stayed put, including the one with the hen in a box. About 15 minutes later, the men arrived back on board, and the bus spluttered its way on. A couple of miles further on, we pulled into another village, the bus stopped, and the men disappeared while we sat, completely confused and a little amused. We were the only non-locals on the bus.

At the third village, curiosity got the better of us, so we decided to disembark with the men and see where they were going. There was a murmur from the señoras in black as the two Irish hussies followed the boys into the local bodega, where they smoked a cigarette, had a shot of some local brew, spat on the floor, and gurgled away in guttural Spanish. We had a quick cortado coffee, a little disappointed that we hadn't uncovered some illegal or at least unorthodox activity.

The bus continued to make its leisurely progress and, as we climbed higher, we reached into our bags for our sweaters. The sky was blue, and the air was crisp as Mount Teide wore her year-round collar of snow. We gazed out the grimy windows at the volcanic lunar landscape just below the crater of this mountain, Spain's highest.

Soon we were descending, and the stops on this leg of the journey were the normal bus kind – picking up and dropping off passengers. We drove through pine forests above the clouds, finally sinking down into the Orotava Valley as darkness fell. We rounded yet another bend, and I caught my first glimpse of Puerto de la Cruz: her flickering lights reflected in the water of the Atlantic Ocean.

As we reached the banana plantations on the outskirts of the town, I had the oddest feeling that I was home. We had come from the south of Tenerife, which is barren, dusty, and desert-like. It gets the best weather, with lots of sunshine and little rain. The north is a different world.

It's lush, tropical and much older than the purpose-built resorts of the south. I was eighteen years old the day when I stepped off that old bus in Puerto de la Cruz. I remember breathing in the cool air; something deep inside me recognised this place as somewhere very special.

Over the following years, Puerto de la Cruz became my second home, refuge, and holiday haven. Working in the travel business, I was able to fly south to this island town in the Atlantic Ocean, off the coast of West Africa, at least once or sometimes twice a year. Each time my arrival was no less of a homecoming than the first.

The old quarter of Puerto de la Cruz is a maze of narrow streets and alleyways onto which a cascade of rapid-fire Spanish falls from various competing TVs. The alleys are punctuated by doorways where women in aprons perch on kitchen chairs, chatting in that dramatic way Spaniards do, which often makes it look like they are gunning for a row. It is a town of tiny shaded squares with ancient fountains bubbling in the sun and the Plaza del Charco, where families gather in the evenings after a paseo on San Telmo. Anyway, you get the picture.

Back in the '80s, the town was still buzzing with life and romance. Nowadays, it has become a retirement town where many old hotels offer "all-in" packages so that many restaurants and bars are quiet and empty early.

However, it is still somewhere I love to visit because it contains a part of my soul. It's a town where I feel entirely comfortable and where I know I could spend months at a time. It is a town that holds part of my history. Puerto de la Cruz was the first place I actively wondered what it would be like to live abroad. I imagined a little house with a garden where I could grow bananas, oranges and lemons. I would learn to speak fluent Spanish and enjoy balmy evenings reading and, of course, writing. Because all my favourite places would clearly unlock my award-winning inner writer.

## Casperia

So, who doesn't dream of Italy? The food, the landscapes, the culture, the language, and the beautiful people. My obsession with Spain obscured the delights of Italy until relatively recently: until September 2008, to be exact.

I had had my first scripts accepted for radio and was more than surprised to find that, along with the privilege of recording them myself for broadcast, I was also paid. Thinking this might never happen again, I opted to blow the lot on a cookery weekend I had seen advertised in Italy. I found a willing accomplice in a friend of mine, and off we went, flying into Rome, from where we made our way by train and taxi, to Casperia, a magical 1,000-year-old village folded into the Sabine hills. We arrived just as the light drained from the pastel sky, painting the old buildings in the warmest hues of soft amber and caramel. I was in love again.

The oldest part of Casperia is walled and consists of narrow, cobbled paths, which wind around the ancient houses. It's stunningly beautiful and a car-free zone. We stayed in a charming B&B, originally a nobleman's house in the village. That first evening we ate a simple meal of pasta, with fresh salad leaves and juicy tomatoes, on a terrace overlooking the rolling countryside watching the changing colours of the sky as the sun slowly sank behind the hills.

The next morning, I opened the shutters on my bedroom window to feast on the view. Below me were laid out rows of terracotta roofs at various angles, beyond which olive groves rose up to pine-clad hills. An ancient tractor put-putted up a lane as it wound its way towards a ramshackle old farmhouse, surrounded by fields of goats, whose bells I had been hearing in my sleep. The air was fresh, and the sky was clear. Swallows swooped and dived only feet in front of me. I breathed in deeply.

Our first cookery lesson was on Saturday morning in a small school a little distance from the village. As we worked in the large kitchen, the resident family of cats wandered in and out looking for scraps. The dogs were sprawled just outside the door, asleep in the autumnal sunshine. The whole experience was sublimely relaxing and akin to being at your granny's in the country. We retired to a long table under a lemon tree in the garden, with ever-hopeful cats winding their way around our legs as we sipped our wine and consumed the delicious results of our morning's work. It was a fine way to spend a

Saturday afternoon. Then we did it all again in a different school on Sunday.

I did not want to leave Casperia with its intoxicating, quintessential Italian combination of languidness and sensuality. It is a timeless place where I could imagine spending days and hours just relaxing and soaking up its energy. And once again, I wondered who Barbara might be if she could escape for a month or two to Casperia or some similar Italian town, experimenting with making pasta and eating lots of tiramisu, living a slow, delicious life in the Italian hills.

## *Perth, Western Australia*

I didn't go to college. I don't regret missing out on "the college experience" and all the "wildness" that entails, but I do sometimes envy students who have the privilege of sitting listening to the brightest minds articulating ideas on a subject that they are passionately interested in. And yes, I know it's never too late, and I could apply to do a degree as a mature student, but that is usually only a passing thought.

Australia was not a country on my list of places I really wanted to visit. I always thought it was a barren country full of surfer dudes, tin huts, sheep, and kangaroos. Yeah, I know. That's like describing Ireland as a misty, rainy place full of leprechauns and dancing girls at the crossroads.

Then my eldest flew south and landed on its western coast, and when I visited a year later, I was blown away to discover that not only was Perth a beautiful city on a huge waterfront, but the country is also much more exotic than I had thought. We had just arrived and were still in the airport car park when flashes of colour in the sky caught my eye... parrots. All over the place. Parrots. In Perth. Who knew? Not me.

Although my daughter lives there, it was not somewhere I expected to consider living until the day we drove past the University of WA, a few miles from the city. As I admired its elegance, I began to wonder about taking a year out to come to Australia and study writing at this lovely university on the water.

I now have two grandchildren in Australia, so I visit more frequently; each time, I reconnect with what I call in my head "my Aussie Granny self". Because my Aussie Granny self is a mature, healthy, strong, barefooted, long-skirt-wearing hippie. And she is directly connected with my fifteen-year-old self, whose hippie tendencies briefly came to the fore. Each time I get to Western Australia, I look forward to my reunion with her, as well as the much more substantive reunion with my girl and her lovely family.

I may never become any of these alternative Barbaras, but that's not the point. The point is that daydreams open our minds to new possibilities, new horizons, new experiences. It makes us believe that the seemingly impossible may, in fact, be possible if we really want it.

# DREAMS OF HOME

For all my fantasies about living abroad, I love Ireland. I know that because I give out about it regularly. I have spent a lot of the past decade talking and writing about how frustrated I get with this place that I call home. Much of what frustrates me can be traced back to bad policy decisions or no decisions at all and a very peculiar system of political parties here.

We have an ancient, rich culture, but we are a very young state, given that we only managed to gain our freedom back one hundred years ago; perhaps there is still an immaturity to Irish politics that doesn't always serve the people well. What has made me angry and frustrated, especially in the last two decades, is our narrowed focus on the economy, with everything else taking very much a back seat. The constant focus on measuring our success as a nation only in terms of economic growth means that social problems become some kind of unavoidable collateral damage.

But Ireland, with all its chronic problems, is home. I love the fact that we love books and writers. I love the fact that we have some of the most incredible landscapes. Most of all, I love our attitude to life. Our sense of the ridiculous. Our humour. And our ability to embrace change.

Despite the freedom that comes with this stage of life and the fact that, as a citizen of the EU, I have the option to move to somewhere better organised, more equal, and warmer, I don't see myself doing that for any longer than a few months. My soul is as dysfunctional as this country, and we need each other.

So, my long term dreams are located right here, here on this little island in the North Atlantic with our winter storms and our underwhelming summers when we can plan nothing due to the vagaries of our mad weather.

## *Peace and Quiet.*

I never noticed the noise associated with city and suburban living until about ten years ago. Overnight I seemed to become hyper-aware of sirens, the constant general traffic hum, and house alarms, and it began to irritate me. Anytime I leave Dublin, for a few days "down the country", hitting the open road begins with a distinct feeling of leaving the stresses and the incessant noise of daily living within my county's borders. As soon as we hit Kildare, Wicklow or Meath, my shoulders drop, and I relax into a different version of myself. Once, that is, I get beyond the thoughts in my head of "did I turn off the heating?" or "did I leave a light on downstairs?" and so on.

Increasingly I am drawn to places where I can be close to nature, places where I can hear the birds singing and feel the wind in the trees and the awe of seeing the universe spread over my head at night. A more rural life would also allow me to indulge in my passion for living with more animals than is practical in the city. Currently, I live with four (sometimes five – long story) cats and one lunatic young Labrador. We also have a squirrel who visits the garden regularly, called Hamlet and Gary the Fox, who arrives every night for his supper.

As I have aged, my love of animals and wildlife has grown, as my irritation with noise increases. I can feel myself growing closer to nature. I wonder what it would be like to have a rescue donkey or two. Maybe have some hens. And a goat or a sheep. Or even a cow. Have you ever stood at the gate of a field of cows and had a chat with them? They have the most amazing eyes. They are curious. And they like music. Yes, I know what you are thinking, and yes, you may be right, but surely eccentricity is one of the joys of getting older and caring way less.

Anyway, I daydream a lot about life in the country, even though I am aware that I may not manage to live for any length of time without the convenience of the suburbs, where everything is within shouting distance. But I wonder how it might be to spend my days pottering about growing flowers and vegetables and chatting with my donkeys.

## Living On An Island

One of the most frustrating things about living in Ireland is the peculiarities of our weather. Although we do have fairly well defined seasons, which I love, we also have weather that changes in a matter of hours. We have to be ready for all weather-related eventualities and can plan nothing without a plan B, the rain plan, even in summer. We take nothing for granted. It makes us a people who can be very spontaneous and open to change.

There is one type of weather here I hate, and it's one we have too often: the grey days, which can often stretch into grey weeks when the sky is on the floor. Days when there is no wind, when everything is becalmed in grey nothingness. The only active thing might be a drizzle of rain. It's the kind of weather that makes your hair frizzy and your brain hurt. The temperature is likely to be somewhere between 7 and 12 degrees. It creates a colourless world that is neither particularly warm nor cold. Bland days that wreck your head when too many come together.

I love a good winter storm when gales lash the house and the downpour comes in all directions. I love the sound of rain pounding the roof and windows and the wind howling down the chimney. I love our skies which move and morph into a myriad of colours and shapes, especially in winter. There is nowhere I prefer to be than West Cork in summer when the sun is baking the landscape under a blue sky reflected in a calm cerulean sea. I would not enjoy living in a country where the weather was always the same – even if that meant blue sky every day.

Outside of the bland grey days, our weather is generally fairly energetic, and I often feel that living an urban life means that we don't fully experience our climate's variety, so I have another dream. And this is one I would love to be able to make a reality.

This dream is of living on one of our offshore islands for a year. On an island, I could really experience a winter storm. I could watch closely for signs of spring's arrival, bask like a shark in the hum of summer, and enjoy an authentic Irish Halloween. I would rent a cosy and warm cottage with an open fire and a spare bedroom so that family could visit. I would take the dog and maybe adopt a kitten. I would write about my adventure and, best of all, I might finally polish up my spoken Irish, assuming that my island getaway was a Gaelthact island. This is something I wish I had dared to do when the kids were young. Imagine the experience they would have had, in a tiny school, learning Irish by osmosis and surrounded by all that wildness.

## ACTIVISM

If all this dreaming sounds too calm and too passive for you, there is one other thing that I think older women can be very good at, and that's activism. As I've already said, we have the time, the space in our heads, and the energy, and once we stop caring as much about what people think, we may find it easier to be "difficult".

As I turn 60, there is one thing that I am sure of (along with lots of things I used to be sure of but which

I now doubt), and it's this. The world we have created (well, let's be honest, the world men have created) isn't great for equality or quality of life. It is also killing our planet. We are at a critical moment when actions must be taken now to have any hope of undoing the damage. As Greta says, "we don't have a planet B".

I think that women, and especially older women, have a real role to play in changing the world. There is a very particular (or maybe peculiar) energy that exists in a room when women gather, be it a group of friends, a book club, or a professional women's gathering. And this energy can change our world. I am sure some clever people might be able to explain the difference, but to me, it feels like something powerful, but softly powerful as opposed to aggressively so. It can often be underestimated, which is where the real power comes from.

Let me tell you a story.

Back in the mid-1970s, when I was about eight or nine, there was a laneway at the end of our road. It linked our estate with the main road into our local town. A developer had bought the land immediately around this laneway, and he had begun to build houses. That was fine except that the local women, many of whom cycled daily to the shops, realised that their laneway was going to become someone's back garden and be lost forever. So, they mounted a simple campaign in a bid to protect this vital access.

They wrote letters to local politicians and to the developer pleading their case. They were clear that a right of way had been established, but no one seemed to be willing to enforce it. Direct action was needed, so their children were primed to raise the alarm if it looked like the laneway was about to be blocked off.

No one expected this work to be undertaken on a late summer evening, but that's what happened. A large digger made its way to the corner of the site to lay waste to the precious laneway. The kids, including me, raced home to tell our mothers what was happening. And the women – only a handful of them – made their way down to confront the workmen. The developer, sensing that there might be trouble, had arrived on site too.

The women stood their ground in front of the entrance to the laneway, claiming it for the community and refusing to allow the digger to proceed. The developer told the driver to go ahead. It was very tense. I remember thinking how brave or perhaps mental my mother was. Standing side by side with her neighbours and friends, she refused to move. The digger driver hesitated before he got out of his cab, saying he wouldn't drive his machine towards a group of women. The women said they would remain at the site all night if necessary. The standoff went on, and darkness fell. There were no dinners that night.

Finally, the developer capitulated. The lane was saved. And I got my first experience of direct action and how it can work, even against all the odds.

The lane remains to this day. Every time I cycle it, I am grateful to those women, including my mother, for their courage and energy in making a stand for their community and what was right.

History is littered with bigger examples of women coming together to effect change. Greenham Common was a mammoth undertaking by a small group of women in 1981, which became a mass movement and moved hearts and minds against nuclear arms. In Northern Ireland, throughout the bloody years known as 'the Troubles,' many groups of women were involved in the often dangerous cross-community work of building peace. The best known of these "peace" women were Mairead Corrigan and Betty Williams, who received the Nobel Peace Prize for their work.

In 1975 in Iceland, 90% of women went on strike for equality, downing tools, whether in the workplace or at home. Again, it moved hearts and minds; Iceland elected the first female head of state ever in 1980 and is still one of the countries closest to achieving gender equality.

In Ireland in 1971, a group of women (members of the Irish Women's Liberation Movement) took the train to Belfast to buy condoms, which they waved about on their arrival back in Dublin, drawing global attention to the fact that contraception wasn't available in Ireland at the time.

Parenting a child can change you and make you softer. It opens your heart so that you become a kind of universal mother, feeling not only your own child's pain but every child's pain. I think a similar thing happens when you become a grandmother. Suddenly your worry about the planet becomes more acute as you become deeply concerned about what kind of planet your grandchildren inherit. Perhaps this is one of the reasons we have grandchildren. It makes us realise that we have a vested interest in ensuring that they have all the opportunities possible and that the world we leave them is at least as beautiful as the one into which we were born.

Women have also traditionally been associated with nature. Our cycles are that of the moon, and, almost as importantly, we know the value in being able to spot a good drying day (yeah, yeah, I know men put out the washing too... some of them... sometimes). Our homes are human habitats, traditionally looked after and organised by women. Caring and nurturing connect us with the creatures with whom we share this planet.

During the second wave of feminism in the USA in the 1970s, a branch of feminism emerged called Eco Feminism. Eco Feminism links the subjugation of women with the need to control and manage the natural world. The patriarchy has traditionally viewed both women and nature as chaotic, unruly and in need of control. So, as women rise (slowly, oh so slowly) to equality, we have a duty of care to change the ways humans treat this planet and all its species. We know that women are more affected by climate change and the natural disasters it causes, so we all have a role to play in the huge cultural shift necessary to protect wildlife and their habitats, biodiversity and welfare.

You don't have to join a group, organise a campaign or chain yourself to any railings (although if you do decide to do any of the above, I applaud you... loudly); you can just use your voice to call things out that are clearly inappropriate or wrong. You can also teach your grandkids and nieces/nephews about the importance of honouring the Earth, caring for the animals and being aware of biodiversity and habitat protection, along with all the other messages about living in a "greener" way.

I wear a bracelet with a tiny elephant on my wrist. I wear it every day to remind me that about three years ago, I made a firm commitment to speak up for animals every time I felt that their welfare was being compromised. My bracelet is also a reminder of a dark day when I accidentally found myself watching a horse race.

I had always been unsure about horse racing and so never had any interest in attending a race meeting, even though I live a few kilometres from one of the country's best-known racetracks. However, I was at Ireland's premier racetrack, The Curragh, in County Kildare on this particular day. I worked with my photographer husband at a very fancy social event. The photography should have been done, and we should have been able to leave before the races had started. Needless to say, things ran late, and we were still there as the first race got underway. The hospitality suite we were working in had a bird's eye view of the finish line. I happened to look out as the horses charged past us, and one fell. It looked like he just fell over his feet. Down he went. The jockey came off, but, unlike the horse, he got up and walked away. I watched, horrified as the horse struggled to get up. I couldn't believe what I was witnessing. I felt physically sick. The horse was clearly extremely distressed. I was horrified and afraid I would vomit, so I went to the bathroom to compose myself. When I got back to the hospitality suite, a tent was erected around the horse, who became another casualty of our horse racing industry. I looked around the room, full of people sipping champagne in their Sunday best, and wondered how no one else was at all put out at what was unfolding outside. I was furious and deeply upset.

I subsequently did some research, which horrified me. Over 120 racehorses died in Ireland in 2019, and the figure for the UK for the same year is 186. We get all dressed up in our fanciest clothes to watch horses running for their lives, a process that often ends in one or more of their deaths. This is entertainment? I will continue to speak up about this cruelty hidden in plain sight whenever I can. And my little bracelet, which Sherwood bought me later that awful day, reminds me of the commitment I made.

Life after menopause offers women a wonderful opportunity to make an impact – this can be just on your own life or in a wider context, perhaps within your community, like my mother and her pals, or even on a national or world stage. Contrary to what the patriarchy might tell us, we only reach our prime when we are post-menopause. This is the time when we are most dangerous and potentially troublesome. Why? Because we have a ton of life experience, we care less about how we are judged. We no longer need the validation we may have sought in our earlier years.

Activism isn't for everyone; I know that. However, as we will explore in a later chapter, learning to use your voice is important whether you use it just within your own circles or further afield. Don't underestimate how much fun you might get from becoming a troublesome woman, aka a pain in the arse of the patriarchy.

## CREATIVITY

Whether you choose activism or not, how many of us have harboured dreams of creativity for years? How many of us have visualised ourselves writing away for hours, putting our ideas, thoughts, or stories down in print? Or perhaps you imagine yourself painting... in a sunny room with an easel and a palette of paint with the freedom to create whatever you wish.

After decades spent living, whatever way your life panned out, it makes perfect sense to me that once you reach your sixties, you are now in an ideal place to experiment with your creative side, even if it is something you have not exercised since you were a child. You have stories to tell, songs to sing, scenes to paint. You have so much experience: a kaleidoscope of life events that you can now use in all manner of creative ways.

So, what exactly is creativity? Creativity is simply about creating something that didn't exist before you brought it into being. Creativity is another way to express yourself, as you do in the way you dress. It's another way to reveal who you are to the world. So, by definition, we are all creative beings.

If you think you "don't have a creative bone in your body," think back to when you were a child. Did you own crayons? Did you colour in? Later, as a teenager, did you doodle all over your textbooks? Yep. You did. All kids do. But something dulls our innate creativity, perhaps during education, or maybe later, when we realise how much of what we do is judged by the world. We apply ourselves to what we deem ourselves to be good at, and we forget the simple joy of doodling or messing with paints. Simultaneously we become our own critics, and if we don't feel our creations are good enough, we abandon the project and, along with it, the many health benefits – both physical and mental – of creative endeavours.

We live in an era of increasing stress, in a world where we think that being busy is a positive. Thus, even if we accept we have a creative side, many believe that we don't have the time to be creative. We may have carved out time for the gym or a walk, but how could we possibly have time to draw, paint, bake a cake or write a story? We have often spent years thinking that mucking about with creativity is something we perhaps hope to do when we retire. Well, the time is nigh, and creativity is good for us.

Creativity relieves stress. If you are engaged in creation, you must be fully present in the moment and be fully aware of what you are doing. This calms the monkey mind that fires all kinds of baloney around your consciousness all the time. Creativity allows us to turn back on our heads while engaging in writing, baking, painting, or whatever. It allows us to feel a sense of achievement and feel calm. We know stress is bad for us, and there is no doubt that it plays a role in many of today's major diseases. This is the number one reason we should all play with creativity.

But there's more. Do you know that even just observing creativity, maybe watching an artist at work or just admiring the work in an art gallery or at a concert can also relieve stress?

Creativity is also good for your brain. According to a study by the Mayo Clinic, creativity may have a protective effect on neurons. Neurons are the basic building blocks of the brain and nervous system. So, in protecting them, creative endeavour may help us ward off Alzheimer's, other types of dementia and other degenerative diseases. (American Academy of Neurology 2015).

Just as exercise can release happy endorphins, creativity can also lift one's mood. You enter an almost zen-like state when absorbed in a creative project, and out of the calm comes increased self-esteem, confidence, and a feeling of peace. In fact, The British Journal of OTs studied 3,000 knitters and found a significant relationship between knitting frequency and feeling content.

Creativity can improve your social life. Many creative endeavours are solitary, such as writing or painting. However, many painters and writers will also join a group to improve their skills and receive feedback on their creations. So you need not be a lonely creative.

Painting is one of the most expressive art forms, and it can be as simple as putting paint on canvas. Colours, shapes, and textures can create a magical work of art, although that's not the only point.

I once had to experience an art session for a feature I was writing, and I was dreading it, thinking I would be the eejit who would produce something similar to my children's artwork that used to adorn my fridge when they were in infant classes. But you know what? I swirled and curled paint in a most pleasing fashion and had the best two hours. It was right up there with having a pampering massage at a spa. Seriously. The result was a bit... well... chaotic. But the process was amazing. And that is the point and the benefit of creativity. It's not so much about the end result as it is about enjoying the process.

Writing is my thing; much like exercise, the more I do it, the more I want to do it. Writing is how I make sense of my world. It's often how I process world or national events. Emotional events also result in my vomiting my emotions into a journal. So, if you feel the urge, write.

If you have a story to share, why not consider setting up a blog? It is where I started trying to get my writing read.

Did you make up stories for your kids when they were young? I did. I loved plundering my imagination with the freedom that only writing for kids gives you. So, if you have stories you used to tell your kids, why not write them down. Your grandkids might love them. Start now if you always wanted to give writing a novel a shot. Don't put it off.

I think I might go slowly mad if I didn't write.

However, you don't have to write or paint to be creative. Cooking, baking and indeed gardening are all expressions of our natural creativity. Creativity has no rules and no limits. And there are so many creative things that you could experiment with – photography, woodwork, metalwork, sewing, knitting, dancing, acting, music, aromatherapy... the list really is endless. I have a friend who uses natural products to create fabulous creams, oils, soaps, and potions. Creativity is freedom. The best thing of all... the more you indulge in creative expression, the more you want to.

Since I was quite young, one of my dreams has been to write a book. However, it's only in the last few years that I have seriously tried to do so. My main problem is my attention span, which is only marginally longer than that of a goldfish. I have started many books and failed to get beyond 10,000 words or thereabouts. However, coronavirus, lockdown and the lack of other work to do delivered me an opportunity to push through, and so, here we are. I seem to have written a book.

At best, dreams can be a launching point for change. To grow, one has to dream. You cannot effect change if you cannot visualise it. As I get older, I have found that I regularly need to interrogate myself about what I want now. How do I want to live? The clock never stops ticking, and I still have so much stuff to do, things to achieve, places to visit, people to meet, and things to make. But each and every one of those things begin with a dream, a visual concept.

So never think that daydreaming is a waste of time. It's not. It's a rich, enjoyable way to begin the path to something new. Even if your dreams don't ever materialise, you will rarely regret succumbing to the magical world of your imagination.

Dream on, sisters, dream big and dream small but dream on. However, if you are to make the most of these delicious years and chase your dreams, be they big or small, you need to have the energy and good health required. By your fifties, you have quite a few miles on the clock. And the chances are that there will be things that need attention paying to them.

# HEALTH

*"Ageing is not lost youth but a new stage of opportunity."*

**Betty Friedan**

## HAPPY FATTY

I wasn't always fat. I wasn't a fat kid. In fact, as I have already discussed at length, I am tall, so I was a beanpole kid: taller than everyone in my class right the way through school. I have always been taller than my friends and colleagues. I was called big, even when I was just tall. "Oh, you're a big girl" is not something you enjoy hearing as a girl, even if you are tall.

Obviously, I was in secondary school when I reached my zenith of six feet. In my bright green uniform of the local convent girls' school, I was the original "Jolly Green Giant". My height guaranteed that I always sat at the very back of the classroom, where I couldn't obscure anyone else's view of the blackboard. I stuck out like the proverbial sore thumb, which also guaranteed that I got caught whenever I was involved in nefarious activities in school. I loved a bit of anarchy but wasn't very good at it as I was like a lighthouse directing teachers to my misdeeds.

This all meant that I learned that I stood out early on and was out of sync with my peers. So, I have always been outside the norm body wise. Thus it wasn't a great culture shock to become fat as the years progressed. However, as I became fat, I also became increasingly unfit. Exercise was never something I enjoyed, another thing that perhaps started in secondary school when, being head and shoulders above the rest, I rapidly came to the attention of the PE teacher.

I was press-ganged into the basketball team from my first year and, as I have already told you, I wasn't a happy or particularly good player. I was an awkward beanpole marooned on a team of serious sportswomen who took every match very seriously.

Of course, the PE Teacher also thought that height equalled muscles, so she signed me up for athletics one year. She was well aware that I couldn't run, so she decided that I was our school's answer to the huge Russian women who were the only shot putters I ever saw. Thankfully, I was even more useless at shotput than basketball. Ditto long jump. So my dalliance with athletics was only one season long.

I lived in fear and dread of PE day being wet, which meant, instead of being outdoors practising basketball or perhaps playing rounders, we were in the "gym" doing the 1970s version of a workout. And I should say that the gym in our school was the hall and the equipment consisted of benches, a horse, and some mats. So, for a tall, self-conscious girl who could never ever even do a forward roll, let alone a handstand or cartwheel (kids in the '70s were obsessed with handstands and cartwheels for some reason), a rainy gym day was a disaster. Secondary school definitely cemented my hatred of sport, which I have carried proudly into adulthood. I don't even watch sport. The only time I ever watched football was in 1990 because that was when Ireland nearly won the World Cup (we didn't – but we might as well have given the excitement of getting into the quarter-finals generated).

# THE WEIGHTY YEARS

My weight was fairly static during my 20s, but giving up fags, in my mid-30s, was the beginning of my slide into eventual disaster. If you grew up in the late '60s/ early '70s, you might also have spent quite a lot of time forcing yourself to like smoking. Smoking was cool. And in a country that was anything but, we all took to smoking like mad yokes altogether. I think it made us feel normal in a land where the Catholic Church was all over everything deemed fun or cool. I don't remember them lecturing us about kids smoking, though.

Back in the mid-70s, it was possible to go into a shop and buy one cigarette. Yep, one cigarette. Shopkeepers were happy to break open a packet of the cheapest fags around (which were called Gold Bond) to sell to the local kids. Can you imagine – a child (I was thirteen, although my height did mean I was often assumed to be older) being able to buy one cigarette? If the shopkeeper was nice, they might even give you a match. One match, which you carefully stashed on your person until you found a safe place, out of the wind and out of possible sight of your parents. There, you would strike the match off a wall and light your one Gold Bond, which was often shared with a pal or two. Inhaling the poison initially made you feel nauseous. Still, it transported you to Paris or Madrid or somewhere where the sun shone. The people were fabulously sophisticated, even though we were sheltering from the wind behind the wall of the local soap factory, which was somewhat devoid of Parisian chic.

Getting the smell of nicotine off your fingers before you went home for your tea was the main problem with this undercover, furtive smoking. Toothpaste was my remedy of choice, although I don't know why my parents never wondered why I arrived at the tea table (we ate dinner in the middle of the day back then) smelling of spearmint.

I didn't take up serious smoking until I left school and began to earn the money that would enable me to buy a whole packet of cigarettes. I progressed to smoking Rothmans, which we used to say proudly back then, "would rip the throat off ya". But if smoking was cool, having a whole packet of fags on your person was the actual height of sophistication. So, I smoked everywhere. Even though neither of my parents smoked, my brothers and I all did, and eventually, we did so at home. Why the parents tolerated their kids turning their lovely "magnolia" walls a light shade of brown is a bit of a mystery, but they did.

Back then, smoking was tolerated in a way that seems daft now. I smoked at work, where I sold holidays over the counter of a travel agency, often through a fug of smoke I smoked a cigarette before I got out of bed in the morning, and last thing at night, I smoked on the bus (upstairs), on flights (beyond row 12 or thereabouts), and I even smoked between courses in a restaurant. That was how cool I was. I smoked through my pregnancy. Yes, I know. Not one bit cool. I am ashamed of that. But, in my defence, my doctor told me to cut them down as we were both smoking at his desk – I kid you not. He said that cutting them out would probably make me a nervous wreck, which would be worse for the baby. But if I limited myself to ten a day, that would do. I know. I know…

Anyway, karma is a bitch and all that, and by my mid-thirties, all that smoking was beginning to catch up with me. Colds turned into bronchitis every single time. And bronchitis robs you of your ability to breathe properly, gifts you a horrible mucousy cough and just makes you feel wiped out. I think it was the third time I presented at my GP with bronchitis that he told me that I should either give up smoking or look forward to some serious ill-health.

Giving up smoking was one of the hardest things I have ever done. Nicotine addiction is very difficult to break. Like all addicts, I always had to have another packet of cigarettes bought before I had smoked the final five in a packet. So, in preparation for giving up, I would smoke all my stock, sometimes one after another, in a vain attempt to make myself sick of smoking, literally. It never worked; without my fags I was grumpy, irritable, and sad. I would struggle through the weeks, congratulating myself every day that I didn't smoke, but invariably on a bad day at the office or a boozy night out, I would succumb. And once I smoked just one cigarette, I was back in the game.

It took three attempts before I was finally successful. In that last attempt, I didn't smoke all my stock. I threw out whatever fags I had left. I made an appointment with my dentist to have my teeth cleaned. And, at the beginning of every week, I took the money that I would have spent on cigarettes, and I bought myself something nice. It helped, but it was still hard. One of the hardest things was having a cup of tea or a chat on the phone without a fag. So, I developed a liking for buns and cakes.

I remember thinking very clearly that even if I put on some weight, I could deal with that once I conquered my love of smoking. Because I reasoned that losing weight would be far easier than cutting nicotine out of my life. I later found that logic to be deeply flawed.

I got married in my mid-thirties and, other than a little baby pouch of a tummy, my lumpy knees, my big feet and sticky-out ears, I was reasonably happy with how I looked, well, as far as any woman ever truly is. In another effort to be cool, I decided that the white bridal look wasn't for me, so I went for red. Bright, scarlet red. My inspiration was Paula Yates, who I had always thought was so cool; she also wore bright red for her wedding to Bob Geldof in 1986. The design of my dress was Grecian, so my look on the day earned me the moniker of "Mighty Aphrodite". This was a definite improvement on the nickname one of my darling brothers christened me with when I was a teenager: "H", short for heifer! And that was long before I actually was a heifer.

By the time I had given birth twice more in my thirties, my weight had begun its upward trajectory. Then I retired from paid work to be at home with my kids and found that I loved being a "housewife" even if I hated that term, and, best of all, I discovered the sublime joy of baking.

Baking, what can I tell you? It is the ultimate magic. The alchemy of turning a basin of slop into the lightest and most sublime sponge is nothing short of miraculous. Now please don't think I am Ireland's answer to Mary

Berry because I most certainly am not. My repertoire is limited enough, but I can make great scones, a decent Victoria Sponge, a very lemony drizzle cake, banana bread, curranty buns and a mean pear and chocolate cake. There is still nothing I find as relaxing as baking. It is the most wonderful stress buster. If I am feeling frazzled, I find the process of baking profoundly grounding and relaxing – all that beating and mixing. And once the ingredients are mixed and in the oven, my kitchen is wrapped in the most glorious aroma, which whispers words like home, safety, comfort, and love. There is nothing like taking a batch of scones out of the oven and letting them cool slightly while you whip some cream and make coffee.

I became the witch I had long wanted to be in the kitchen. Baking is something that is something deeply rooted in our female bones. It is something our mothers, grandmothers, and great grandmothers did. It is intrinsically linked with providing care and love to your family. It is the one thing that really does make me feel like a domestic goddess in a way that cleaning the bathroom or washing tons of clothes doesn't.

The only downside (and it wasn't a downside until recently) is that I am my own baking's biggest fan. I joyfully munched my way through most of what I baked. But I felt like such an earth mother when I always had a little homemade something to offer visitors with their cuppa. When *The Great British Bake Off* began on telly, I was in heaven. I will admit that early on in series one,

I became so enraptured by the baking on screen that I paused the telly to go into the kitchen and make a chocolate cake so I could enjoy a large slice with the rest of the episode.

Of course, I was a sucker for home baking elsewhere too. My favourite cafés were ones where the coffee was good, but the baked goods were sublime. I rated all the local supermarkets based on their bakery. Mornings weren't mornings if they weren't punctuated with a coffee and scone break. I loved my treats. And if I didn't have some of my own in the kitchen, I would sometimes send himself off to pick up some pastries for our coffee, something he was happy to do.

I don't want you to think that I sat and scoffed cake all day. I didn't. But food was my go-to comfort. A bad day meant that I didn't want to cook, so we would "treat" ourselves with a take out. And Fridays were always take-out night because who the hell wanted to cook on a Friday? In fact, I had a long list of days on which I decided I wasn't cooking.

Every Friday, they included my birthday, International Women's Day, Mother's Day, Nollaig na mBan and all bank holidays. Bear in mind that it is only relatively recently that one could order a reasonably healthy take-out meal. Most of the takeouts in my life have come from the local Chinese or the chipper. I am not blaming either fine establishment for my malaise, though; my issue was how often we ordered them. For my wedding, my darling mother wrote a poem which she gaily recited at the reception; it included a reference to how worried the local Chinese takeaway were as they feared that my getting married might mean I moved house, in which case they would likely go bust.

And guess what? Big surprise… all this contentment meant my weight slowly crept up. But Goddesses are voluptuous. I was finally the big girl I had been called since my childhood. OK, there were times when I was shopping for an outfit for a special occasion, and I would get mildly frustrated with trying to find something that didn't make me look like a sack of badly packed potatoes. But so what? I can genuinely say I wasn't that bothered. I had been called "H" for so long that, in some ways, being fat felt a bit like coming home, not as a large female cow but as the cuddly, furry, round Mama Bear I always knew I was.

## BODY POSITIVE

As a feminist and someone who still passionately believed in being body positive, I felt very strongly that my rotund appearance was a testament to the fact that I wasn't a shallow woman (in every sense of the word) who was overly concerned with my appearance. Oh no, my jelly belly was evidence that I was happy and content and had no fucks to give. I was far more concerned with real issues than I was wondering if my bum looked big in this. (It always did. So what?)

I still think that. How we look is no one's business but our own. In fact, as a mother of daughters, I have spent hours lecturing them on how there is far more to them than how they look. I have pointed out to them all how society delivers really horrible messages to young women (and increasingly to young men too now) about how they should look and what is acceptable and what is not.

What I missed, though, until it started to smack me in the face, was that I was increasingly unfit. I once had a friend who used to tell me that my problem was that I loved myself too much. She didn't mean it as an insult but a closely observed appraisal. And I always thought she was right. Most of the time, I do like myself or even love myself. I like to do what makes me happy when I can. For the last two decades, a lot of what made me happy was retiring to the sofa when the work of the day was done (and I do work hard) and putting my feet up, with a cuppa and a slice of cake or ice cream or whatever sweet treat took my fancy. I hibernate very well. Mama Bear again.

Of course, along with treating myself to delicious, tasty bites to eat, I was just not moving anywhere near as much as I should have been to keep healthy. When I was in school, being forced into all kinds of physical activity, walking to and from school, and using public transport, I was reasonably active. When I left school, I began to work in the city, and my commute involved a 20-minute walk to the train and another ten-minute walk from the station to my office. So, I walked for at least thirty minutes per day without even trying, which didn't include a wander down and around town on my lunch hour. It also didn't include the amount of walking we did at the weekend. Not hiking in the hills but walking home from late-night movies at 2am or just from the pub. We regularly walked two or three miles home without even thinking about it. A taxi was an unaffordable luxury back then.

But over the years, my activity levels got less and less. I learned to drive. I had the money for taxis. I didn't need to walk if I didn't want to. Having young kids does keep you on your feet, but you blink, and they are teenagers. (OK, –that's a lie – it's a long, exhausting process). Then they don't need you running around after them anymore. You are consigned to merely being a cook and a chauffeur. So, after ten years at home being a housewife and baking myself into bliss, I reinvented myself as a writer. Yep, it's a great job when you are fat and lazy. It involves sitting on your expanding arse for hours on end, attempting to be creative, something you believe is much helped by cuppas and chocolate.

## EIGHTEEN STONE AND UNFIT

I first began to suffer from migraine when I was in my mid-thirties. I was working full-time and had small kids. Life was busy and, at times, very stressful. At the time, I wouldn't have thought I suffered from stress. Exhaustion, yes. But stress? Not so much. Then I realised that many of my migraines landed immediately after a particularly busy time at work.

Migraines are not just headaches. They are mega headaches accompanied by other wonderful side effects such as disturbed vision, nausea, and sometimes vomiting. The pain is indescribably intense. When I get a bad migraine, I am rendered completely useless. I can't sleep, I can't relax. I wander from bed to bathroom to kitchen, seeking relief.

Once I realised these early migraines were stress-related, I began using meditation, breathing and making largely unsuccessful attempts to calm my monkey mind. However, once I left the world of paid work to "work" at home with my kids, bad as it could be on a rainy day, it was far less stressful, so my migraines lessened considerably.

During menopause, they returned and were exacerbated by alcohol, as I've mentioned.

Giving up the drink was not as hard as the cigarettes, but it was still hard. I didn't think I drank a lot until the day I was at the GP for something or other, and he asked me if I drank much. No, I said not much. How much he asked. A glass or maybe two (it was always two and sometimes even three), I said. "A week?" he asked. I looked at her to check if he was joking. He wasn't. No, I said, a night. Oh, he said, clearly nonplussed, that's quite a bit. I wasn't sure whether I should have been proud or worried.

Of course, once people heard I was giving up my red wine, I was assured that the weight would fall off me. Someone told me that a glass of red wine was the same as a doughnut. Great, I thought as I waited for the weight to drop. It didn't. Not one pound did I lose, which led me to think that God, in her infinite wisdom, had clearly decided that I should be fat.

Around the same time as I broke up with my beloved red wine, I decided to become a vegetarian. In fairness, I was never a big red meat eater. I grew up with a mother who would have taken a bite out of a lamb's leg if the lamb stopped for long enough near her. She loved her meat. She loved bloody meat. I have memories of coming home after Sunday Mass at about noon; she would open the oven where she had beef roasting and slice off a piece to have with her cuppa. It would be red raw. It horrified me. And she is as much of an animal lover as I am. There was a time when I loved a bacon sandwich. I loved charred cocktail sausages. I even loved the odd, very well-done burger. However, by my fifties, the only meat I was eating was minced beef and chicken.

My youngest turned vegetarian when she was about 16, and so a year later, myself and himself decided to give it a go too. Once I thought about it, I hated knowing that what I was eating was once a live, breathing animal. It was the easiest "giving up" of all. I am a very happy vegetarian. Veganism is on the horizon, although I do love my dairy, so I currently live in the hope that we can work out how to produce butter and cream without tearing baby cows away from their mammies.

The point is that although I was clearly overweight, I kind of felt that I was reasonably healthy. No alcohol and a meat-free diet with lots of vegetables and fruit. I was fat, but so what? I was rarely sick, except for migraines, and I prided myself that I was on no long-term medications by my late fifties.

There was, however, an elephant in the room. And I don't just mean me. The other elephant was my complete lack of fitness.

Although I denied it for a few years, I was getting breathless too easily. I avoided stairs because I had to stop to catch my breath too often. My knees started to act up, as was one of my ankles. I avoided low chairs and sofas because getting out of them was initially very ungraceful and subsequently nearly impossible. I love a bath, but getting out of a bath was getting trickier due to my weight and the fact that my poor knees were under enormous pressure. I had a technique that worked at home, but it could be an issue when staying in a hotel. In fact, I very nearly got stuck in a bathtub in Copenhagen a few years ago.

Flying was always a worry because I was right at the limit of the seat belt's length. The next step was a belt extension. My mother told me at one point that I waddled rather than walked, which kind of stunned me, but I knew she was right.

There were things that I would have liked to do but wouldn't or couldn't because of my weight. My daughter was home from Australia a few years ago, and we had a family weekend away in the beautiful Parknasilla in Co Kerry. On the last morning, we had arranged to go kayaking to visit some seal colonies. When we got down to the water, we were given life jackets and, yes, you've guessed it, mine wouldn't fit. I immediately took it off and laughed it off. "Too fat for kayaking anyway," I said and, in my head, knew that I would have looked ridiculous anyway. My daughters were unhappy as they really wanted me to be part of this family adventure. "I'm fine," I lied, "sure I'd frighten the seals anyway. I'd look like an elephant on an ironing board coming towards them." And leaving them laughing, I made my way back to the hotel. On the way, I met the kayaking boss with whom I had booked our trip.

"Where are you going?"

"Back to the hotel to wait."

"Why?"

"I am too fat for the life jackets".

"Don't be daft. They expand"

And he marched me back to the water where a jacket was expanded to fit me, and off I went with my girls. A very grateful elephant on an ironing board. It was a sublime experience and one I will remember forever. I could cry when I think of how near I came to missing out on it altogether.

Spas are another horror when you are fat. It is mortifying to undress, only to find that your robe doesn't come near to closing. You get dressed again and make your way to reception to report the problem, which the hotel or spa may or may not be able to solve for you. I know it shouldn't be mortifying, but it is. After it happened the first time, I phoned ahead each time I had a spa booking (which wasn't that often) to request a size 20 robe. Sometimes it worked. Sometimes it didn't, and I ended up in a robe that more or less closed, as long as I didn't sit down. The other problem was rolling over on the narrow massage table without falling off. Not easy when you are wide as the table and not particularly agile.

When I became a grandmother at 55, I vowed to work hard to have a real relationship with my adored granddaughter (and, latterly, my grandson), even though they live 11,000 miles away. Long haul flying requires stamina and reasonably good health, especially when you are doing it regularly. So I knew I should do something about getting fitter. I did not want to be an unfit granny who couldn't do anything active with my grandchildren. Despite my lack of fitness, the travel went well until we got hit by a global pandemic, which has literally grounded us.

So a few years ago, I did make a real effort to lose weight and regain some functioning level of fitness. With the help of a wonderful personal trainer, I managed to lose about half a stone. But once I achieved the weight loss, some madness in my brain told me, "sure, you know you can lose weight, so no pressure; have the cake, you can lose it afterwards." I like to think I am a reasonably intelligent woman. In fact, I am an idiot. I have a great relationship with my grandkids, but even so, the arrival of my precious granddaughter was not in the end enough for me to take my appalling level of fitness seriously.

Every so often, I would think, "I will start walking every day". But my knees didn't like that, and then I developed plantar fasciitis (horrible heel pain), so inevitably, I would walk for a week or so and then give up as my legs and feet were sore. And back came that voice in my head who loves me to tell me that clearly, God wants you to be fat. "You are fine as you are," it says, "sure, have the slice of cake."

Then I got very tired. Very, very tired. Let me explain.

# JULY 2019

West Cork is not so much a place as a state of mind. I have found my own personal paradise on the Sheep's Head Peninsula, which I visit every summer for a week or maybe two. It is a perfect place to rest, reset the internal dials and just breathe. Because time is different there. It's slower. The days are languid and filled with the heady scent of honeysuckle, fuchsia, and montbretia overlaid with the tang of the ocean. It's a place full of rambling boreens and tiny lanes at rise and fall, lost in oceans of dense fern where velvet and suede cows meander over to the gate to stop and stare at me with their deep, soft, dark eyes. The nights are black as melted tar and more silent than you could imagine possible. It is a balm for the soul, a perfect counterpoint to the busy lives we all lead. It's a place to rest, just be, read, write and think. I know. I can't describe the beauty of the place without becoming a wee bit poetic. West Cork is where I go to renew my sanity every summer; I return, if not quite a new woman, certainly a revived one.

The summer of 2019 was a particularly busy one. The Australian branch had been home not just once but twice. They first arrived in late March, just as spring was bursting forth all over the place, and stayed for three weeks liberally sprinkled with some good weather. This trip had been planned for over a year. We visited the zoo, the playground, and the park and took lazy, slow walks. We went out for brunches and lunches and spent the evening fussing over my granddaughter as we bathed her and read her bedtime stories before tucking her in for the night, after which we all chatted for hours. It was a lovely time.

They returned again in July for a wedding in Italy; this time, I got to look after my granddaughter for five days while her mum and dad went to the wedding. Before they went, we had an early second birthday party in the garden and filled the time once again with days out and just hanging out together. I loved every minute and cherished the memories we made together, but I had forgotten how full-on having charge of a two-year-old is.

Saying goodbye is always hard, especially when you are unsure when the next visit will be. It's something you never get used to, which always leaves me emotionally drained. So, by the time they left, I was totally out of battery. But I had West Cork, and this time we were staying for ten whole days, after which I knew I would be revived and back to full charge again.

The feeling of anticipation and freedom as you hit the road in summer for your own favourite part of this wonderfully beautiful country is delicious. And although the weather wasn't brilliant, we all soon settled into West Cork time.

Every year, we book the same house; it is located a few minutes' walk from the tiny village. It is on a slight hill, so it also has the most glorious view over the quaintly named Kitchen Cove, its tiny little harbour. I had brought my laptop, so I could write. I always feel that I will be inspired to write beautiful prose there, the kind of writing I dream of being able to create, which might be inspired by all the beauty and silence. I had also arrived loaded with books and music.

My husband is a photographer, so he amuses himself by trying to capture some of what makes the Sheep's Head so special; our youngest, who has also fallen under the spell of the place, likes to paint. As well as pursuing our various creative activities, our days are also spent walking, drinking coffee, and eating cake (of course) in the café of dreams in the village. Honestly, I can't explain how perfect these days are. They are complemented by nights spent in a tiny tin-roofed pub chatting to locals and just enjoying time out of life.

We feel like we are nearly locals ourselves, and this familiarity adds hugely to the holistic benefits of our time there. I can usually feel myself being steadily recalibrated.

However, in 2019 my batteries wouldn't recharge. Every time I sat down to read, I almost fell asleep. One night I couldn't even move myself to go to the pub. It didn't worry me until we were into our second week, and I was still feeling as exhausted as I had when we arrived. I knew that this wasn't right. If West Cork couldn't revive me, well, clearly nothing could. I thought there might be something wrong.

A few nights after we came back to Dublin, I lay in bed and started to google why I might be exhausted all the time.

# AUGUST 2019

Let me say now that when you are an aul wan of 57, you think everything that ails you, from migraine to exhaustion, is due to menopause. I thought this might be another gift that goes with being a woman. We are so used to our lives being ruled by our hormones. But Google disagreed. When I asked it why I could be tired all the time as a somewhat overweight woman in her fifties, it wasn't menopause that came up. The top answer to my question was actually Type 2 Diabetes.

My heart sank as I delved deeper.

As usual, I look for the Irish answers and here is what I found from the Diabetes Ireland website.

You are more at risk of getting Type 2 Diabetes if you are:

- Over 40 years of age. *Yep, I was fifty-seven.*

- Have a parent or brother/sister with diabetes. *Yep – my dad developed type 2 diabetes in his fifties*

- Had diabetes during pregnancy. *No*

- Are overweight for your height. *Oh Yes*

- Do not take 30 minutes of physical activity daily. *Yep, that's me*

- Have high blood pressure. *No, my doctor has remarked before that I have blood pressure I don't deserve.*

- Have high cholesterol. *Not that I knew of.*

You may also have Type 2 Diabetes if you recognise any of these symptoms:

- Blurred vision. *Well, I have been wearing glasses since my mid-30s*

- Fatigue, lack of energy. *Oh, a major yes.*

- Extreme thirst. *When I gave up alcohol, I consciously tried to drink more water. I was convinced that some of my migraines might be due to dehydration. So, I always have water with me. So, I guess that's a yes.*

- Frequent trips to the bathroom (urination), especially at night. *Well yeah... but the water. My husband had prostate cancer, so he goes in the night and sometimes wakes me up. And then I go. Not together, you understand... I mean, seriously?*

- Rapid and unexplained weight gain or loss. *Mmmm... dunno about this one. Never experienced much in the way of weight loss ever, even when I was trying. And my weight gain was fairly well explained.*

- Frequent infections or a slow-healing sore. *No*

- Numbness, pain or tingling in your hands or feet. *Yes, I had recently had numbness in one finger.*

Further searches revealed other risk factors, including yeast infections (I had recently had one, something I hadn't had for ages) and big babies – I am a big woman, so naturally, I had big babies.

By the time I had turned off the light to go to sleep, I knew I had diabetes. I wasn't shocked, but on the edges of my consciousness was the realisation that I wasn't as clever as I had thought I was. Because this was my own doing. I had known I wasn't fit. I had known I was overweight, but I had not been concerned. It seemed as if I was right, that all that was about to change.

# DIAGNOSIS

The next morning, I made an appointment to see my GP. My GP is a lovely man, but (thankfully) not someone I see (thankfully) that often. However, following the sudden death of a friend who was just a few years older than me, I had had a full medical early in 2018, and everything came back fairly normal. Of course, my dear doctor did give had given me the lecture about losing weight, and I did give my standard response of, "'Yeah, yeah, I know. I will get to it. Soon''. And here I was, just 18 months later. I told him that Dr Google and I thought I had diabetes. The doc was very sceptical. I told him about the exhaustion, but he thought it was likely something else as my blood sugars hadn't been abnormally high at my relatively recent medical.

However, he did a blood sugar test on the spot, which changed his mind and announced that I might be right. To properly diagnose diabetes, you need a particular blood test called an HbA1c test, which measures your blood sugar levels over the previous three months. So, I left a sample with him and waited to hear my fate. Sure enough, a few days later, I got the call to tell me that yes, I was now a diabetic, and an appointment was made for me to come in and talk to the nurse at the practice.

I can't say I was shocked. My fate was, I guess, inevitable, although I had been in denial. For years, I had been a diabetic waiting to happen. My overwhelming feeling at my diagnosis was one of disappointment in myself. My cheerful refusal to accept reality had led to this point. And I had a fair insight into what was ahead, even before speaking to the practice nurse.

As I mentioned already, my father was diabetic. He was diagnosed in his mid-50s too, and initially, he was put on insulin injections. This was back in the '70s, before the internet. I remember my mother going to the library to get all the books she could, to know which foods he could have and which he could not.

I am far more like my mother than my father. A quiet, conservative man of routine who was happy to stay home. He liked peace and quiet. He was a civil servant all his working life and took his job and life much more seriously than Mother. My mother is a bit of a nutter with a parenting style that was, as I have already alluded to, let's say… interesting. Suffice to say, my mother loved the craic, and it took precedence over housework and domesticity. So, her learning about food choices in the '70s had been as steep a learning curve for her as it was about to be for me, four decades later.

Back then, my dad's new diet had featured a lot of salads. And sugar-free chocolate and jam because my dad loved his cake as much as I did. In fairness to him, though, he did take his diagnosis very seriously. The fact that he lost a big toe to his diabetes might have helped focus his mind. Although I am assuming that he had been diabetic for longer than before he was diagnosed.

Along with his new diet, the most dramatic thing he did was buy a bike. This was long before "mamils" (middle-aged men in lycra), cycle lanes, or cycling was considered cool. In the '70s, my dad, the self-described "senior civil servant", started to cycle to work every day. He worked in the city, and we lived in the suburbs, so it was a cycle of ten km each way. But maddest of all was the fact that he came home for lunch. Yep, he cycled a 20 km round trip to have lunch at home. He must have had very long lunch breaks. I also remember, well after he retired, that he cycled to the airport and back one day. That would be a distance of over 40 km.

He had to inject insulin twice a day when he was first diagnosed. A year or so later, he managed to switch to oral insulin. Another year or so further down the road, he controlled his diabetes through a good diet and daily exercise. It's funny, but we children weren't that bothered when he was coming to terms with his diabetes. We were busy teenagers, and, as long as he seemed to be alright, we weren't concerned or even that interested in how he was adjusting to his new lifestyle.

But now, my dad, who died in 2002, is often on my mind. I remember how serious he was about taking control of his diabetes. Two decades after his death, it is his stoicism and determination that I draw on, taking not just comfort but also motivation from him. My ole dad, the man with whom I had so little in common, is now my role model. That inspiration began when I decided to take this threat to my health seriously and begin what I had put off for years and years... losing some weight and getting fitter.

I fully expected that all the support I would need for this radical lifestyle change would come my way. However, a week or so after diagnosis, I realised that this was not the case.

I left my doctor's surgery after a motivational, reassuring chat. I was also given a phone number for the Health Service (HSE), who would link me in with their community workshop for newly diagnosed Type 2 Diabetics. They would provide me with all the information and support I would need. So far, so good.

I immediately called the number, dying to get started, only to be told that the next workshop in my area was at the end of October. And it wasn't really in my area or on a bus route. I would need to drive to get there. I wondered how newly diagnosed diabetics who didn't have a car would manage. Remember too that this was mid-August. And although I wasn't that surprised at my diagnosis, it was a shock to know that I now had a life-changing condition, which was potentially serious. Thanks to my dad, I knew I could control it, but I just didn't know how. I did know that I had to act while still in mild shock at the initial diagnosis. I have enough miles on my clock to know myself well. I knew that if I waited two and a half months, I would have convinced myself, sure wasn't I fine, and once again, I would have prevaricated about making the changes that I had long known were necessary for my general health, well before diabetes arrived to deliver me a sharp kick in my not insubstantial ass. But it seemed I was on my own. As usual in Ireland, the community health service is a great idea, which isn't always fully realised.

Everyone knows the obvious first step; I had to ditch the sugar. I have already mentioned how I loved to bake and how I prided myself on often having some class of home-baked goods in my kitchen. All that had to go. My stock of cake was fed to the birds in the garden. Like when I gave up cigarettes, I knew I was best going cold turkey.

I stopped always having ice cream in the freezer. I got rid of my favourite blackberry jam. I donated my chocolate stash, which wasn't huge in fairness because a little chocolate went a long way with me. However, I always needed to know there was some chocolate because, when I needed it, I NEEDED IT.

I am not going to lie; it did feel bleak. Here I was, a non-drinker, a vegetarian and now I was also the "I am trying to lose weight and I am diabetic" gal too. I was going to be great fun to go to dinner with.

"Em, do you have a vegetarian menu?"

"Just water for me, thanks."

"No dessert, thanks, just coffee."

I am cheap, though, that's for sure.

I had never even taken regular vitamins. But now

I was diabetic, I apparently needed to take something called Metformin which was to help my body deal with glucose, of which there was too much in my blood.

A few days later, I was back at the clinic to see the practice nurse who ran Diabetic Support. We had a good old chat, which focussed mainly on losing weight and strategies for that. I also left with another prescription, this time for a statin, because my doc had decided that my cholesterol was a bit on the high side. Now I had two tablets to take every day. I suddenly felt old and a bit crocked. I also had the problem that I had very difficulty remembering to take either tablet – never mind both.

Two weeks after diagnosis, I hit the wall. Well, the first wall. This was as the realisation of the reality of being left to fend for myself set in. I began to spend hours online, researching the best diets for vegetarian diabetics who need to lose weight. I found fasting diets, keto diets, low carb diets and many apps and programmes to follow if you download a yoke onto your phone. I was literally drowning in information, some of which was contradictory. After a few days of this, I broke down in tears sobbing to myself, muttering that all I wanted to know was what I could have for my bloody lunch. Or dinner. Or breakfast. To say I was confused and frustrated was an understatement.

By nature, I am an over-sharer. My life is generally an open book, and nothing is sacred. I used to work in close proximity with a lovely man who is still a great friend, but I freaked him out on average once a week by asking him questions that he considered to be completely off-limits. The day I asked him if he had a vasectomy, he nearly fell off the chair. I had only been being a good wife and trying to do some research for my husband, who was contemplating the snip. Anyway, I share. So my instinct was to widely share the earth-shattering and totally unsurprising news that I was now a diabetic. Although, if I am being honest, my motivation was somewhat selfish. I know I have enough ego to not want to fail publicly. So, if I talked about how I now HAD to lose weight and get fitter along with overhauling my diet, there was a much greater chance that I might succeed.

I am an avid user of Twitter and Instagram, so I began there. As any regular user of these platforms will know, you will get all kinds of advice thrown at you when you decide to share personal information. Most of it is well-meaning. Some of it is purely commercial. Some of it is completely wacky. Some things were useful, but I knew I had to find my own way through this from the get-go. I had to come up with a routine that worked for me. I politely acknowledged and thanked everyone who threw all kinds of information in my direction. However, can I say that the general support and caring I found online was a huge help to me. I found it very reassuring and still do. The online community is often painted as aggressive, cruel and mean, but there is another side to it that I happily participate in. And like life itself, there are far nicer, kind, funny people online than nutters.

Anyway, my online witterings led to me doing a bi-monthly column in a national newspaper charting my journey, as well as many radio interviews. A friend of mine heard one of the latter. This good friend was also a diabetic and a nurse. She called me and, sensing my frustration, did what all good nurses do – gave me clear instructions. Get on the phone to your GP, she said, and get yourself referred to the Diabetic Unit in my local hospital. So simple. It is still a mystery why no one mentioned this to me.

I got a referral and had an appointment a couple of weeks later.

Before that, however, I got the fright of my life. Something that shook me far more than the diagnosis itself did. Something that shook me to my core.

I was driving with my middle daughter not far from home on roads I knew well. I have been short-sighted since my mid-thirties, which means I have to wear glasses for driving, watching TV and when I am out and about. As we turned a corner, we came upon road works with a myriad of signage for various diversions, and I suddenly realised I couldn't read them. "What does that say," I asked my only glasses-wearing daughter, who had no such problem. Later that night, when I was sitting watching TV, another activity for which I needed my glasses. I kept taking them off and wondering why they were smudged and causing my view of what was happening on-screen to be blurry.

"My glasses have stopped working," I said to himself. I couldn't see with them, and obviously, I can't see without them. This was on a Sunday night, about two weeks after diagnosis. Two weeks after cutting sugar abruptly from my diet. I knew that diabetes could affect your eyesight. I decided I clearly had some kind of rapid diabetes that had already affected my eyesight. What terrified me was that I went from being able to see (with my glasses) to not being able to see either with or without them, literally over a weekend.

Off I went to consult with Dr Google again. I looked for an explanation as to what could be happening to me so suddenly. Could it be the medication? With Dr Google, you will often find confirmation of whatever mad idea you have in your head. Brexit and Trump are both results of people having their biases confirmed by the internet. However, even knowing that, my research concluded that it was the statins. I stopped taking them.

The following morning, I called my GP and told him the story. Fine, he said, stay off them for a week, see if your eyesight improves and keep me posted. Then he called me back about five minutes later, saying that I also had to get myself to an optician as soon as possible and get checked out. I could have had a bleed behind my eye.

Now I know all about bleeds behind the eye. My mother suffered from macular degeneration and had numerous bleeds behind her eye. A long story about some botched treatment of the same means that she eventually lost sight in one eye. She operated reasonably well with one. But she was eighty-four. I was fifty-seven, and I wasn't ready to lose sight in even one eye. I was by now convinced that I was heading for serious eyesight issues.

I made an appointment with my opticians for a full bells and whistles test of my eye health. The appointment was for two days later, and I can tell you with my hand on my heart that those two days were among the longest I have ever endured. I was convinced that I was in big trouble.

In the end, my eye health was pronounced excellent. No sign of any bleeds or anything else sinister. This was a huge relief, but when had my sight tested, the results stunned me altogether. My optician announced that my eyesight had improved... by about 50%. I felt like Lazarus rising from the nearly blind. I can see. I can see. Better than before. I still need glasses but only milder ones now. This was great news. I was relieved and thrilled to bits. I thought that this might be a gift from my body for giving up sugar. My body was saying, "Well done, we like this less sticky blood and so we can operate your eyes better, so carry on."

Unfortunately, it also meant that I had to get new glasses and new sunglasses ASAP. So, €350 lighter, I bounced out of the shop feeling entirely smug. Sad to say, the improvement was short-lived. A few weeks later, I was back in the opticians having the lenses replaced again as my eyesight settled back to what it had been for decades.

The whole episode took me to the depths of terror, but it ultimately made me feel that my body responded to the new lifestyle that I was beginning to implement. It thus gave me the impetus to carry on just when I needed it most, and I went back on my statins.

# A CHANGE OF LIFE

*"It ain't over till the fat lady's fit."*

**Anon... (or maybe me)**

I was diagnosed with Diabetes in mid-August 2019. After a few weeks of intense frustration while I tried to come to terms with losing weight along with cutting sugar from my diet, I began to get a handle on what to do. But it wasn't easy.

## LOSING WEIGHT

We live in the information age, and while that is largely empowering, it can also result in getting overwhelmed by the amount of contradictory advice and help out there. However, I discovered two things early on that helped me hugely.

One is that eating healthily is not as complicated as I initially thought. Like many overweight, unfit people,

I had spent years avoiding information about calories, fats, balancing food groups and other head-melting stuff. When confronted by this stuff on TV or whatever, my brain went "la la la" while I moved my fat ass to find the remote and turn off this offensive stuff that was assaulting my ears and my brain. Having avoided all such talk for years, I not only didn't have a clue, but I also had a powerful instinct to avoid engaging with it. I had to overcome this mental block, but when I did, I discovered that, like much in life, it wasn't half as complicated as I had thought it might be.

At the Diabetic Clinic, I got a copy of the food pyramid, which was helpful. Even the most health-resistant of us know that we need to cut carbs, cakes and unnecessary snacking and eat lots of fruit and vegetables. However, diabetics, we need to be careful of fruit as most fruits are remarkably high in fruit sugars.

The second thing I learned quickly was that I had to establish a routine that worked for me. There is no point in slavishly following a diet plan if it contains stuff you don't like. I had to find a low calorie, no sugar, vegetarian plan. I soon realised that I could find stuff that appealed to me and fit all my criteria by combining various diets. This is important because it allows you to take full responsibility for your weight loss. If you farm out the task to a third party, you can blame them if it doesn't yield results. So, if you want to lose weight, don't be a slave to what worked for someone else. Find food and recipes that fit your particular criteria and compile them yourself to have a range of "go-to" meals that you like. As I often said in those first few months of my new lifestyle, in the end, it all boils down to what the hell you can have for breakfast/lunch/dinner.

For me, breakfast was the hardest nut to crack. Up until Diabetes, my "healthy" breakfast was a bowl of Special K, with a sliced banana and low-fat milk, or, sometimes in summer, a smoothie full of summer fruits. But the sugar content of most cereals ruled them out, and the fruit in my smoothie was also too high in sugar. It took weeks of experimenting with all kinds of stuff, from Greek yoghurt to granola and back again before I hit on something that I like. Overnight oats soaked in low-fat milk and a spoonful or two of no-fat yoghurt, which I combine with mashed banana and heat in the microwave. Not only do I like the taste, but the oats also keep me from feeling hungry mid-morning.

Another huge issue for me, the blame for which I lay totally at the feet of my brothers, with whom I shared my childhood, was portion size. My portions were American-sized and then some. In fairness to my brothers, it may not have been their fault. They did hoover up large quantities of food when we were young, and I was in perpetual fear of there being none left for me. However, maybe it is cultural or cellular memory of the famine that meant that I thought caring for myself and my family meant producing large quantities of food. I loved having leftovers because they often provided lunch the next day. In essence, this had meant that I could eat two dinners a day – a leftover one at lunchtime and then my regular dinner in the evening.

The portions of carbs, usually pasta, rice or potato, had been the main problem of Diabetes and weight. You probably know this, but if you have also been in denial, let me tell you that carbs provide energy, and we need them in our diet; when we eat too much and don't move enough, carbs are converted into sugar. So, they are a ticking Diabetes bomb if, like me, you eat too much of them and like your sofa too much. So I began to weigh out my portions to control my natural urge to put on enough for everyone (which was too much anyway) and then some more just in case. In case of what, I don't know. Anyway, cutting down on portions, especially carbs, was possibly the biggest single change I made to how I eat.

Snacking, especially in the evenings, was something that took all my willpower to overcome. I was a big fan of dessert, an hour or so after dinner. My TV snacks of choice were something from the cake tin or a serving of ice cream. But they had to go. That was hard. Very hard. I found one particular type of apple that I loved. Combined with a spoonful of peanut butter, I found a very acceptable snack. I also keep a small stock of dark chocolate for those moments when only chocolate will do. Two squares are acceptable and enough to calm the chocolate craving.

I was also given a sugar monitor by the Diabetic Clinic, a vital tool in helping me to understand what foods were problematic and to monitor my progress. It functions like a tell-tale friend. One night, I scoffed at half a bar of milk chocolate in the dark in the utility room because I thought that if no one saw me, it didn't happen. The next morning, my blood sugar monitor roared my weakness as it proclaimed (to me and the diabetic nurse I sent weekly reports to) that I had fallen off the wagon. I loved my blood sugar monitor.

I should also mention that with the blessing of the diabetic nurse, I came of metformin as I was determined to control my Diabetes by changing my diet and lifestyle myself.

## Hibernation

A few weeks into my new regime, autumn arrived. Dark evenings, dropping temperatures, and the first of the winter storms all carry one message – stay indoors, stay cosy and just relax. In other words, revert to Mama Bear and hibernate. Autumn is also the season of comfort food, cottage pies, bangers and mash and crumbles with lashings of custard. And just when you think the season couldn't be any more wonderful, along comes Halloween, bringing with it jumbo bags of sweets and chocolate. Autumn is my favourite season.

Naturally, I panicked. Because I knew I had to change my view of autumn. Just like my life, it needed an overhaul, which is difficult to realise you loved things the way they were. It's like having one of those celebrity home makeover people arrive into your home to tell you that your beloved kitchen has to go because it's in danger of destroying your whole house as it's not structurally sound.

My panic was combined with that old voice in my head, the one that had scuppered any previous attempts at losing weight by saying things like "oh sure go on, one cake won't hurt" or "you've been great but now it's time for a treat". Now, I am all for treats when there is a state occasion, but the three months of autumn in all their fabulousness isn't one.

And that right there is one of the biggest challenges I have faced in attempting a lifestyle change: overcoming my unhelpful mind; the inner voice which tells me "it's too hard", "it's not worth it", and best of all, "I deserve a treat". Getting into some kind of weird argument in one's head is a waste of time and energy. The best way to counter this voice was to tell it to shut up and that I was no longer listening. A wise teacher once told me, "you are not your mind." So I learned to hang on, telling the voice in my head to shut up and that, like a marathon runner, I just had to keep on going.

There was an unexpected bonus before any appreciable weight loss, albeit rather mortifying. My shopping bill came down by about €25- €30 per week. I was never one for buying lots of treats (I baked, remember), so this saving was due to the reduction is in the quantity of food I was buying, especially butter.

I never realised I used so much butter. Saving in the region of €100 per month has meant that I can indulge myself with something nice, like a massage or a facial, for example. And that's my treat right there, as I tell my mind. It was nearly as good as a warm scone, oozing melting butter under a generous dollop of tart blackcurrant jam. Not quite, but nearly. I mention scones a lot. I still miss them. They are reserved for special occasions now.

In the end, I negotiated that first diabetic autumn reasonably well. The next thing to test my mettle was a holiday. In Ireland, 2019 was a fairly dismal summer. I love the sun and am a firm believer in the health benefits of vitamin D. So, as we hadn't been abroad that summer, myself and himself took ourselves off to my beloved Puerto De La Cruz in Tenerife for some relaxation before winter kicked in.

I carefully chose a hotel that was a little out of town in the hope that my exercise regime would continue organically as we walked into town at least once a day. I also took my blood sugar monitor with me so I wouldn't be tempted to throw sugar caution to the wind.

Flying from Dublin to the Canary Islands takes about four and a half hours, so it pays to plan if you are trying to control what you eat. Airline food is never great, and on short-haul routes, much of what is offered is packaged up with other stuff in "meal deals". For example, I wanted some cheese and crackers, but I couldn't buy them on their own, as they were part of a "deal" that included chocolate, crisps and shortbread. I settled on Pringles (not great). We bought a salad at the airport to take on board with us on the way back.

You will be glad to hear that I am not going to bore you with all the details of my holiday, but I will say that I did a lot of sunbathing, reading, more swimming than I would normally do, and we walked between 5 and 10km every day. This exercise included a ten-minute clamber down many steep steps to the town. Walking is much more natural when you don't have access to a car and don't have to worry about the weather.

Yeah, I hear you mutter, but what about the food? Well, sure, isn't half the point of a holiday being able to eat out every night: lounging at the pool during the day with the only decision to make is where you might eat that night?

But after two months of working hard on my new lifestyle, I was determined that the new me would have to change how I ate on holiday. Now don't get me wrong, we ate out every night, and we ate well, but the days of starters, main course, and dessert with a bottle of wine and drinks at both ends of the meal are over. We generally only ate a main course and dessert was a coffee afterwards. Most nights, our dinner cost less than €40.

I will confess to having a small jug of Sangria most nights because, well, Sangria. And, the joy of joys, I discovered that it didn't give me a headache. On the final night, we decided we might treat ourselves to a dessert because flan (or crème caramel to you) is another delicious Spanish must-have. However, when mine arrived, all I could think of was what it would do to my blood sugars in the morning. So I only ate about a third of it. I might have gone the whole flan had I known that my sugar monitor batteries had died, and so I couldn't take my bloods the following morning anyway.

Our hotel was a lovely family-run establishment whose clientele were mainly German; perhaps that's why our bathroom came with weighing scales. So, the day before we left, having had what I considered a very healthy holiday and feeling good and fitter than I had been in decades, I weighed myself. The scales showed me that I had lost another half a stone since I had last weighed myself (about a week previously). I got on and off three times to ensure they were correct, and I got the same result each time.

I bounced out of the bathroom to share this good news with himself. He congratulated me but urged caution. The scales were the old-fashioned ones, and ours at home are digital. He thought I should wait until we got back to see what our scales said before announcing the result to the world. Of course, he was right. When I got home, I discovered that I was the same weight I had been when we left for the Canaries. So maybe it was the slice of toast at breakfast or the Sangria, which countered all the walking and resulted in my weight remaining static.

Was I disappointed? Yeah, I was a bit. But the real kicker was that himself, who ate as healthily as I did but drank an awful lot of beer and swam hardly at all, had lost three pounds. As my dear mother was fond of saying is, "don't expect life to be fair because it isn't."

## *Midwinter*

I had lost just over a stone by midwinter, and things were motoring along just fine. But I have lived with myself for over 57 years, so I know myself quite well. When things are just fine, I tend to get a bit bored. And when I get bored, I have been known to do something daft, just to relieve the monotony and add a frisson of excitement. Not the most intelligent approach to boredom, I know, but there you are.

In the end, I didn't succumb to my temptation to give it up for a while, and I stuck with my programme. A serious diagnosis helps focus the mind; there is no doubt. Type 2 Diabetes is a serious illness. The wonderful thing about it is that you can control it with an overhaul of your lifestyle. However, left undealt with, it can cause all kinds of problems. It can damage your kidneys, your heart, and your eyesight, and it can cause the loss of a limb as blood flow to your extremities is affected. Unfortunately, because Type 2 Diabetes is so common, we think of it as a rather benign condition. It is absolutely not, and it has to be taken seriously if you don't want permanent damage done to organs. Permanent damage isn't reversible.

Since I began talking publicly about my Diabetes, I have been stunned at the number of people who contacted me about someone they love who won't take their diagnosis seriously and whose health they are worried about. They are right to be worried. I figured that I had been lucky. I got a diagnosis of something that I could positively impact. Imagine if cancer could be treated that way? I have friends who have died of cancer in their late forties and early fifties. I reckoned I was lucky, and I was determined to make amends for the damage I had done to my body because an unhealthy lifestyle generally causes Type 2 Diabetes.

And that leads me on to another unexpected but very real consequence of getting a diagnosis of Type 2 Diabetes, and that's guilt. Yes, guilt. My name is Barbara Scully, and I am guilty of damaging my previously healthy body. And I don't say that to be flippant. Guilt is something I know a lot about; it is a damaging, destructive emotion. It is also the first cousin of that other master of darkness – shame. I loved myself so much that I indulged freely in treats and things that I enjoyed while becoming less and less active.

As you know, I am all about body positivity. I rail against the constant focus on women's bodies so that no matter what we achieve in life, we had better look good while doing it; otherwise, it isn't worth a fig. I rail against the ridiculous and nigh on impossible grooming standards women are expected to adhere to. I hate that, as a woman, you had better not age either because that is another thing that will make you invisible. I call bullshit on all that.

While I still totally support body positivity, it should not overshadow the responsibility we all have to ourselves to remain well and strong, particularly as we get older. I was lucky enough to have been given a healthy, fully functioning body, and the fact is I neglected it. I thought I was being kind to myself. But now I wonder: was I?

Is being lazy being kind to yourself? I knew I was fat. I also knew I was unfit. I also knew that being unfit is unhealthy and is not something you can keep putting off dealing with. Being unfit and fat puts pressure on your body and, in the end, something will give. With my family history of Diabetes, I knew I was more at risk of developing the disease. I am not stupid, but still, I did nothing until I was forced to. I could have avoided this disease. I didn't, so I now owed it to my body to try to put this condition into remission. I am honestly ashamed that it took me so long to take my health seriously.

All through that autumn and winter, I was marooned in a place where I was afraid to bake in case I should "reawaken my inner cake monster" (my daughter's phrase) who might return with a vengeance, singing "come on Barbara, you know that cake tastes much better than skinny feels." Kate Moss was wrong, very wrong. Some things do taste better than skinny feels.

Christmas pudding is one of them. I make great Christmas puddings. Yes, puddings, because I normally make three. One is for my mother, and one is for Christmas Day (although only half will be eaten as my girls hate pudding), and one is for, well, him and me probably. Although, in fairness to him, he usually gets tired of pudding by mid-January, whereas I will happily munch on pudding every evening until Easter if it lasts that long. And there are so many ways to eat pudding – with brandy cream, Baileys-flavoured cream, custard, plain cream, or (best of all) fried in butter. But sometimes, the universe conspires with you, rather than against you and that first diabetic Christmas and my puddings were a fright. They were awful dry yokes, so I decided to bin them before New Year's Eve. Another win for Scully.

By Christmas, I had realised that controlling my monkey mind was the key to changing everything. Just learning to ignore it helped hugely. I never realised just how much time I spent thinking about food until I became healthier. My mind was very focused on food and had been for decades. Trying to change that habit, which is only a habit, was quite exhausting. You are trying to control your urge to eat something delicious but highly calorific while wrestling with your delinquent mind.

For years, I would be thinking about what I could or would eat from when I got up until I went to bed at night. I wondered about breakfast, lunch, and dinner and about snacks at any time. I also treated food as a reward and comfort. Bad day – have cake. Good day – get a takeout because you deserve it. I had to learn to just stop thinking about food. I learned to recognise what I called "a food thought" and just let it go. I finally learned not to engage with it.

In the process, I fell in love with coffee again. In the past, I would rarely have had a lone coffee. My best coffees had always been accompanied by a little something.... and sometimes not so little. It could be my favourite, a scone (you know this), or sometimes a little pastel de nata or any other kind of pastry... but coffee on its own? Nah. But I have changed. I have learned to love my coffee on its own. There is nothing that can beat a hot, strong, flat white.

# GETTING FIT

So far, I have not mentioned exercise. That is because you can't (to coin a phrase) "outrun a bad diet". Losing weight is mainly about what you eat. However, getting fit is where exercise comes in. It is easier to move if you weigh a bit less too.

I have mentioned how unfit I was a few times, and this appalling fitness level was beginning to affect my life – and not in a good way.

Let me count the ways. If we were going to walk to a local restaurant for a meal out with friends – all of whom were fitter than me – I knew I would be breathless and red in the face by the time we arrived. Of course, I would never admit that they were walking too fast for me, and they were too polite to comment on my scarlet face and panting. And that was after a short walk of maybe 10 or 15 minutes.

Steps were a nightmare. Once a week, I went into the city for a radio slot. I parked in a multi-storey car park, and I usually park on the top floor. I fooled myself into thinking I was great if I walked down the stairs, but I always took the lift back up. I could not manage going up more than one flight of stairs without looking and feeling like I was about to have a heart attack.

I love a bath. There is nothing like a long, relaxing soak in an oily bubbly bath. Nothing. My mother (bless her) always said that a good bath could cure everything from a headache to a broken heart. That's patently untrue, but I know where she was coming from. Being able to shut oneself away for an hour while one bathes is sublime. It would be more sublime if we evolved to the point where we no longer thought it was appropriate to have a toilet in a bathroom. Who on earth thought that was a good idea? A man who doesn't bathe, I suspect. The same goes for ensuites. I do not want to have a ringside position and be within earshot of my partner's nocturnal peeing. I like the loo to be at least the width of a landing away. I would be delighted to have the bath in the bedroom, but we have to get toilets out of our bathrooms. Toilets should be in their own room, complete with a small washbasin, because a bathroom should be just that – a room purely for bathing and showering. It is a divine space where one can luxuriate for hours in a beautifully scented bubble bath without being disturbed by someone banging on the door imploring you to hurry up because they need to brush their teeth.

Even worse is when you are preparing for a glorious spa-like bathing experience, and you hear someone rustling a book and locking the bathroom door, indicating a prolonged visit, rendering the room unusable for some time, after which you open the window so that by the time it is, well, pleasant on the nose, it's bloody freezing.

End of rant. Where was I? Oh yeah, baths.

Baths can be difficult to get out of if you are a bit lardy and unfit. As you put on weight, your knees and ankles start to feel the strain, and this can make it almost impossible to haul one's ass out of a bath.

And. of course, there was a myriad of problematic things because I felt too fat to do them. Sitting on the ground – because I would not be able to get up without looking ridiculous. Low chairs and sofas for the same reason. Flimsy looking chairs. Knowing that I was probably taking up more than half the seat on a bus. Oh, the list is endless.

Nothing makes you feel old before your time more than being unfit and fat. Lifestyle change is the only game in town when it comes to managing your (Type 2) Diabetes, and that means not just food but also moving more. Exercise burns those pesky carbs, so moving around – EVERY DAY – was vital if I wanted to make amends for the damage I had done to my body.

Walking seemed to be the obvious exercise for me. No special equipment required. I could do it whenever it suited me, and it was free. So, I began walking. I set myself a target of walking for about 45 minutes a day. I knew if I wanted to burn calories, I had to walk fast, so I did my own version of power walking for about a week before hitting a problem. My poor knees and ankles objected very strongly, so I had to cut walks short and hobble painfully home, upset with myself that I had failed.

I realised that I couldn't rely on walking alone. I needed to do something else. The only other thing that I can do and have enjoyed in the past is swimming. There were a million reasons I had given myself why I couldn't go swimming. Being fat, I wasn't hugely (boom boom) enthusiastic about baring my body at a swimming pool, which I assumed would be full of water nymphs. Then, I had to wash my hair afterwards, which seemed like a huge palaver. I would have to shave my legs and underarms and tackle the old bikini line too. It all seemed like a huge amount of effort, so I hadn't actually been swimming (except on holidays) for years.

I knew our local community leisure centre had a pool, and when I checked their timetable, they had lane swimming at 9 pm, which seemed like a great time. I could let my hair dry naturally, as I would be washing it in the shower in the morning anyway. And I did discover that swimming at night was a nice way to end a day. I actually found it relaxing.

However, do not think it was all wonderful. My appalling level of fitness meant that I struggled up and down the lanes and was breathless and red-faced by the time I made it from one end of the pool to the other. Even in the slow lane, I was overtaken by others. However, during September and October, I swam about twice a week, and while I didn't love it, I did feel good afterwards, and it gave my poor joints a break from my walking struggles.

Once winter kicked in, I abandoned swimming because I was just too cold when I got out of the pool, and I hated coming home with a wet head. So, I decided it might be time to utilise the gym. The gym. Me. Go to the gym. I was terrified to my core at the very idea. Images flooded my brain of my humiliation at not being able to handstand or cartwheel as a kid, coupled with my dread of so-called gym sessions at school. Then there was my conviction that gyms today were likely to be full of fabulous, toned bodies about two or three decades younger than me, working out in the near dark on machines that both physically and metaphorically looked like they were designed to inflict some kind of torture. All of this and the added torture of the assault on my ears of blaring techno music would most likely result in a migraine. No, the gym was not for me. I'd be too out of place there. The mortification would be excruciating. To use a gym, I would have to lose weight and get fit first. I have said it before – I don't think I am a stupid woman when I am an eejit.

Anyway, my options for burning carbs were shrinking, so if I was to spare my knees and ankles, I had no choice but to attend the gym. I phoned the community one, where the pool is and booked a one-to-one session with a personal trainer. To say I was nervous was an understatement. Even though I am well used to being self-deprecating in all manner of situations, I don't relish making a total eejit of myself. I felt fat, unfit, and totally out of place arriving for my session. And there was a loud voice in my head, urging me to get back into the car and drive home. However, the fear of what Diabetes might do if I didn't take control was stronger, and I kept putting one foot in front of the other to the desk where I met my trainer. A lovely young woman who didn't do a double-take or have to smother a laugh when she saw me.

The gym was a surprise. There was a bit of boom-boom music, but it was a bright and airy space. Most surprising, no one paid any attention to me at all, and not everyone there looked like a bodybuilder. It was all very, well, normal. The lovely young woman took me through the machines explaining each one and getting me to do the minimum on each one. Once the relief of not feeling as conspicuous as a pig in a field full of sheep passed, the full extent of my lack of fitness hit me. I was reasonably useless. I did leave mortified. Not because of anyone's judgement but my own.

On my second visit, one of my daughters accompanied me, and I concentrated on just using the cardio machines, in other words, the bike, the rower, the cross trainer (which was a bitch to master – I discovered I have a real lack of coordination between my arms and legs) and the treadmill. As we moved into winter and my swimming decreased, I paid visits about twice a week to the gym. I even took out a membership. Like walking and swimming, I can't say I loved it, but I always felt better for doing a 45-minute workout. And slowly, very slowly, I improved.

Exercise became important in my life, and I learned to make small changes that added more opportunities to move. I tackled those stairs back up to my car in the car park. If I took public transport, I got off a stop early to walk further to get home. If I was taking the car, I deliberately parked further from my destination than I would have previously. In this way, I tried to build walking into my every day.

Wait, I hear you say, I thought walking was a problem because of your knees? It was, but a chance meeting with an expert in health and human performance (no less) changed that. I told him about my problems with "power walking" and my knees and ankles. He said, "Stop power walking and just walk."

In other words, just go at your own pace – and you know what? He was right. Once I slowed down, my knees and ankles didn't complain as much. It's amazing how a small bit of advice can make such a difference. Of course, as I lost weight, the pressure on my joints eased too. Now I can walk for hours without a problem.

In January, six months after diagnosis, I finally had an appointment with a consultant. I knew I had lost almost two stone, and I felt good. Well, except for one thing. One part of my body was unhappy with this newer, fitter me. And that was my hair. Yep, more hair issues.

It started when the back of my head appeared in a video someone shared on Instagram. "There I am," I thought and then, "what's that on my head?" I kept replaying the video and couldn't work it out. Finally, I took a screenshot and maximised it. What I could see was my scalp. MY SCALP? Through my now flimsy curtain of hair.

Now I am normally a glass-half-full woman, and it takes a fair bit to knock me off my perch. But seeing my scalp completely threw me. I cried. Big salty tears. I was delighted that I was fitter and healthier, but was losing my hair a price I was happy to pay? Not really.

Once I dried my tears, I headed for my local pharmacy with my new tale of woe. I came out over €100 lighter, having purchased special wonder shampoo and conditioner along with huge brown tablets – all of which were going to fix my hair. However, the pharmacist did say that my hair had merely had a shock (dropping sugar and all that exercise) and that, once it got over that, it would be back.

The next stop was my patient-beyond-belief hairdressers. I had decided that my shoulder-length hair needed to be cut. Short. A pixie cut. I didn't care about my big sticky-out ears. Seeing them was a darn sight better than my scalp. Once again, they sat me down, got me coffee and calmed me by telling me that, although my hair had got finer (thinner), it wasn't as bad as I was making out. They would cut it to a nice bob and add some highlights to make it appear fuller, and I would be grand.

So, I rocked up to my consultant appointment with my new thin hair and a bag full of nerves. I had done my best to tackle my Diabetes, but I was worried that it wasn't enough and that my sugar levels were too high. Although my blood sugar monitor showed my bloods were in the good range, the HbA1c test might tell a different story because, in the immediate three months before my appointment, there had been both Christmas and my birthday when I had broken a few rules. I hadn't gone mad, but I had indulged in a few desserts.

I was thus unprepared for what the consultant told me.

I had put my Diabetes into remission. Gloria halleluiah. It had all been worth it. My bloods were back in the normal range, so there was more sticky blood doing damage to my organs. I cannot tell you the relief. I didn't worry every day about being diabetic. But I knew that I had been the master of my disaster and had wanted to undo the damage I had caused my body.

Diabetes has given me back so much of what I thought I had lost forever: things I thought I had lost because of my age. Like dreading, you might be asked to sit on the ground because you know you will not get down gracefully and will likely need a hoist to raise you back up again. Now, don't be fooled, I still resemble a particular awkward camel trying to get down onto the floor, but I can do it. I can get up too, if not elegantly. I no longer dread a lift being out of order or arriving at an unfamiliar building to find the person you are meeting is on the third, fourth or fifth floor, and there is no lift so that you will arrive red-faced and breathless.

I would never have made the lifestyle changes I did unless I had been forced to. That is not something I am proud of. But the real truth is that I wasn't as old as I was feeling. I was just unfit.

I couldn't wait for springtime when I might be able to buy some new summer clothes and dispense with my current wardrobe of tent dresses. Little did I know that by the time springtime rolled around, my world (and probably yours too) would shrink to a few kilometres from my front door as we began the long battle with COVID-19. But there was one other long-lasting benefit that being forced to change my lifestyle brought… and one that still brings me great joy and freedom. And it all began with Sheila.

# SHEILA

Two years ago, myself and himself took off for a long weekend to Denmark and Sweden. We had a lovely time visiting the cities of Malmo and Copenhagen. I came home full of admiration for the women of all ages who cycled in both cities. Now, these weren't like the lycra-hugging, ass in the air, slightly maniacal cyclists we are used to seeing here (and who are usually male). No, these were "ordinary" women, who seemed to be cycling to work, to a meeting, to the coffee shop or to do the shopping, dressed in regular clothes. It was their poise and presence as they sat upright on their old-fashioned bicycles, making stately progress through their city that I seriously envied. They were cool, calm, serene and fit and healthy. I wanted to be like them.

I didn't articulate my thoughts out loud to himself, but I thought more than once that if I ever managed to lose weight, I might like to have a bike, a bike just like those cool Scandinavian women.

After my Diabetes diagnosis, I even went so far as going to a bike shop to investigate their "sit up and beg" bikes, but I never got as far as purchasing one. I think I knew myself well enough to fear that I wouldn't use it, and it would remain, an expensive folly, sitting our shed where it would provide luxury accommodation for spiders.

Then the Australians came home for Christmas. In the week before their arrival, my daughter mentioned a few times that they would have a lot of luggage with Christmas presents and have to accommodate Santa's visit here. "So, maybe bring two cars to the airport," she said. Although she works in the travel business, my daughter has no idea how to travel light. Perhaps that's because she lives in Perth, the most isolated city in the world, so if she takes a flight anywhere, it is a longish one. And she hasn't been compelled, sorry, I mean trained, by Ryanair into packing everything you need for a week's holiday into a tiny suitcase. So, when she said to bring two cars, she meant to bring two cars, which we duly did.

There was a lot of luggage as usual, including one enormous box which made my heart sink. I assumed that this was undoubtedly something for the granddaughter, which she would get full use out of for the two weeks she would be here after Christmas, but which will then live in our attic as it would be too big to take home. Our attic is already full of baby equipment and baby clothes.

Christmas morning in our house has always been manic. The first festive season he spent in Ireland, my English husband was gobsmacked at how we conduct ourselves on Christmas morning. And this is nothing to do with kids. We have always done Christmas this way and think, in Ireland. We are not unusual. First thing on Christmas morning, before anyone has had more than a glass of orange juice, all the presents are distributed. Himself said it resembles the first day of the January sales: in the space of about 15 minutes, everyone has a pile of gifts with only the vaguest idea of who gave what to who, and the house is full of oceans of wrapping paper and boxes.

Of course, when our granddaughter is with us, her discovering what Santa has left happens first, and we have the manners to pay attention to all that before the ruck under the Christmas tree. Once it was all over and we were all basking in the glow of Christmas morning, I was told to see what was in the kitchen. There, in the middle of my kitchen, was the most gorgeous, mint green, old fashioned, Dutch-style bike festooned in tinsel. That was what had been in the brown box, and himself had put it together in secret in the shed. Yes, I cried. Only my eldest daughter would think that bringing a bike from Australia to Ireland was even a vague possibility. I was thrilled.

My new bike was so gorgeous that I wondered where she might live. I knew she wasn't going to spend any time in the shed with the spiders. So, she lives in my office, beside my desk, where I can admire her beauty. Her name is Sheila.

We bade the Aussie branch goodbye yet again in early January, and I waited for the weather to settle down before finding out if it was true what they say about riding a bike.

I bought myself a helmet, which apparently goes with Sheila's old-fashioned vibe but makes me look like a geriatric World War One German soldier.

I discovered that, yes, I could remember how to ride a bike. I could balance and move my legs on the pedals for forward propulsion. However, I soon discovered that I had forgotten some of the finer details, such as getting on and off with any, well… not even grace, just efficiency. Getting on, pushing off and starting to pedal in the required direction involves a level of multitasking that initially escaped me. I am sure my efforts much amused the neighbours.

Once I got going, things were not too bad until I realised I had gears. Gears. No one mentioned gears. My childhood bikes never had gears. Do they work on the same basis as my car? You know, second for going uphill and fourth or fifth when cruising along. I decided to assume they did.

My second important discovery was that the world isn't flat. Most roads and cycle tracks may look reasonably level, but they hide secret gradients that only become apparent as your peddling becomes less effective. Lower gears are of limited usefulness when a dodgy fitness level hobbles you, so your progress becomes slower and slower until you realise that you are not going anywhere at all and your bike is actually about to fall over. This forces you to attempt a rather rapid dismount before both you and the bike crash to the ground. To retain some semblance of bike street cred, I try to give the impression that I actually meant to stop, something best achieved by grabbing my phone to answer an imaginary urgent phone call.

In my car, I can parallel park. I can judge the space my car requires quite well. I am fond of muttering to other drivers, "ah here, you could get a double-decker through that gap". But for some reason, judging distance and speed when on my bike was initially a mystery. For example, when cycling on a cycle track, attempting to overtake a family out for a walk, I was never certain that I had enough room to pass them safely and, on occasion, veered into the grass, which tended to throw the steering and balance into chaos. I am still a bit hazy about the etiquette involved in overtaking walkers. Should I ring my bell to announce my approach, or should bell ringing, like beeping the car horn, be reserved for serious situations? Initially, I resorted to muttering loudly, "oh hello, em thank you," as I wobbled past. Now I just zoom past on the grass.

In fact, wobbling was a constant hazard. On my second excursion, I was crossing a road, and there was a little kerb up onto the cycle lane. At the last minute, I decided that "bumping" up onto it might be a mistake, so I executed an urgent swerve and stop accompanied by another inelegant dismount, much to the amusement of passing motorists, I am sure.

Those early days were a bit fraught, and I doubted that I would ever cycle very far on my bike but thought it would provide me with another form of exercise because I still find walking EVERY day can get a bit repetitive even if I don't do the same walk twice in a row.

I was just getting used to the mechanics of cycling, still only along cycle tracks, when the great pandemic of 2020 hit and we were locked down and instructed not to go more than 2km from our homes. The traffic just stopped. Overnight it just melted away. The roads were weirdly quiet. Conversely, the cycle tracks I had been cycling were now full of families with kids and dogs and were harder than ever to negotiate. So, I took to the roads.

Gloria, hallelujah, I was cycling on roads. Proper roads. I was whizzing around roundabouts and sailing through junctions like a proper cyclist... only slower. But, still. And the freedom. On a bike, you tend to explore more. You check out laneways and roads whose destination you have long wondered about; something you wouldn't do walking because if it went nowhere, you'd have to walk back.

More than that, I started to remember shortcuts from my youth. I revisited places I didn't even know I remembered. Shortcuts we used to take, through lanes that only locals know exist. I have shown himself part of our world, in which he has lived for 24 years that he never knew existed.

I guess I was lucky that, as I began to ride my bike, the country went into lockdown, and the roads became incredibly quiet, allowing me to gain confidence much more quickly than I might otherwise have managed. However, if you drive, you already know how roads, lanes and junctions work, and it's not as terrifying as I originally thought. I am cycling more than I had ever thought I would. When I dreamed of getting a bike, I used to think if I could cycle to the local post office or shop would be amazing. Now I am cycling into the city, something I never thought I would or could do. That's a return journey of about 24 km, which I know is not huge in terms of serious cyclists, but this is some achievement for me. The feeling that I have propelled myself into the city under my own steam is wonderful, as is the slightly smug sense that I have done something really positive for the planet by leaving the car at home. The vagaries of Irish weather mean that I don't do this as much as I would like, but I am happy each time I manage it.

We have also begun to explore some of Ireland's wonderful 'greenways' – new cycle trails that usually follow the route of old railways. We have spent long weekends peddling through scenery that would otherwise be hidden. My bike has opened up a whole new world for me.

Sheila is the best thing that has happened to me in years. I love her to bits. I am not quite the elegant Scandinavian, but I am good enough. And although hills are a killer and some are 'get off and push' jobs, cycling downhill with the wind in your thin, grey hair makes you feel like you are ten years old and makes you want to shout "wheeeeee". I think my old dad would be most pleased.

# A WOMAN'S VOICE

*"It took me quite a long time to develop my voice and now that I have it, I'm not going to be silent."*

**Madeleine Albright**

## OUR STORIES MAKE US WHO WE ARE

In the first part of this book, I shared many of my stories from the various decades of my life. I did this because my experiences have made me who I am. They are part of me; they shape my opinions and my worldview. And yours are a huge part of what makes you, you. They are intrinsic to who we are. However, our stories should do more than that. They should be the fuel that drives the national conversation because contained in our stories, in our lived experience, is the latent power to change the world, making it a better place for not only women and girls but for men and boys too. For too long, women have shared their stories only where it has been safe to do so.

From professional networking groups to book clubs, from coffee mornings to weekends away, women are generally very good at talking, really talking, with each other. Deep in our bones, we have an almost primitive understanding of our need to share our stories, experiences, and opinions. For centuries, we have been doing it from the Red Tents of biblical times to women's empowerment events today. Connecting with other women allows us to learn from each other. It helps us make sense of the world and validates our experiences when they are often not valued in the wider world.

However, we are generally not good at taking our conversations, stories, and opinions to a wider audience. We are not great at raising our voices, so they are heard in the town square, in the public space still dominated by the male voice and the male viewpoint. Women have yet to be fully valued in this space.

I remember watching Mary Robinson's acceptance speech on her election as seventh President of Ireland and the first woman to hold the office back in 1990. As she acknowledged those who had voted for her, she said, "…the women of Ireland, mná na hÉireann, who instead of rocking the cradle, rocked the system, and who came out massively to make their mark on the ballot paper and on a new Ireland." I was extremely moved by her words; perhaps that was the first time I really believed that women, with all the lingering inequality our gender still endures, could actually be a force for positive change in Ireland.

Of course, it wasn't the first time women in Ireland had used their voices to push for change. Although I wasn't taught it at school, Countess Markievicz, the first woman elected to the Parliament in Westminster and the first woman minister in the Irish Dail, wasn't the only woman involved in pushing for equal rights and independence in Ireland in the early 20th century. She was part of a generation of women, committed and rebellious feminists, who were effectively silenced by a strongly conservative and Catholic Ireland post-independence, which sought to place women back in the home.

The so-called second wave of feminism took place in Ireland in the 1970s and coincided nicely with our entry to the EU (or EEC as it was known). It resulted in many positive legislative changes, especially supporting lone parents and removing the marriage bar and contraception. Our national conversation was also enhanced by some brilliant outspoken women journalists and broadcasters. However, today's media, especially broadcast media, is still dominated by the male voice.

## A LOUD VOICE

My father, bless him, spent my childhood years telling me I had a voice like a foghorn. He also used to tell me I should be careful, knowing how awkward I was. He was a man who liked his peace and quiet, and I presumably disturbed that regularly with my combination of crashing into things and having a loud voice. I will own the crashing into things, but the loud voice I lay at the feet of my three brothers. I needed my loud voice. Since then, I have often been told that I have no need for phones. People tell me they could probably hear me without the need for any technology at all.

All girls should be encouraged to have a loud voice and use it confidently. Because despite all our progress, women and girls still struggle to be heard. To be taken seriously. To be listened to. This is particularly apparent in boardrooms, where men generally do most of the talking and interrupt women a lot more. A study at George Washington University found that when men talked with women, they interrupted 33% more often than when talking to men. Watch a panel discussion on TV, and you will see the same phenomenon.

Barack Obama's female staffers noticed this problem during his first term of office and came up with a plan to overcome the male domination of meetings. They called it "amplification". One woman would repeat a suggestion made by another woman, giving credit to its originator, thereby ensuring her voice, her idea, and her opinion was heard and was not (as often happens too) hijacked by one of the men. Mary Beard writes of this hijacking of ideas in her excellent little book Women & Power. She reminds us of a Punch cartoon from almost thirty years ago, which depicts a board meeting with one woman and five men. The caption is, "That's an excellent suggestion, Miss Triggs. Perhaps one of the men here would like to make it."

Oh, but how many of us have been Miss Triggs at one time or another?

Things are changing, but far too slowly. There is, however, one forum where women's voices are being heard: social media.

I was an accidental early user of Twitter, which I began to use around the same time as I began to write my blog, From My Kitchen Table. I had always written, from angst-ridden teenage poetry (which was mainly about not being ridden) to resort reports during my first career in the travel business and press releases when I worked as PRO for a national charity. Around the same time, I joined Twitter, I also embarked on a creative writing class to polish my amateur attempts at words that would engage and enthral readers.

I hit a problem that took me literally years to solve early on. I needed to find my writing voice. It kept coming up again and. It took me years to have the confidence not to attempt to emulate other writers I admired and to be myself instead. To write unashamedly as me. The place where I found my voice was on Twitter. Twitter helped me learn that people responded when I was authentically myself. When I tried too hard, they generally didn't.

All of us, writers or not, need to find our own voice. To have the confidence to share our own opinions and experiences. Of course, we also need to listen, but generally, women are more used to listening than speaking publicly.

However, we all know that women also get some of the most appalling abuse and threats on social media and, in general, sadly on Twitter. Some of our best female broadcasters and presenters have left the forum because they couldn't stand the level of abuse hurled at them. However, I think it's vital that women stand their ground on the platform, difficult as that may be. It is too powerful a forum for us to leave it to the bullies and the trolls.

Women have successfully driven movements such as #MeToo and #EverydaySexism on social media platforms, and these campaigns have resulted in some very real change. These seemingly harmless hashtags have allowed women to have their voices heard and to tell deeply personal and disturbing stories of sexual abuse, harassment, and violence. Social media is immediate. There are no gatekeepers to negotiate. Therefore, it can facilitate change in a way that traditional media seems to find more difficult so far.

The power of women's stories cannot be underestimated; the brave cohort of women who told intensely personal stories played a huge role in propelling the movement that resulted in our recent repeal of the eighth amendment allowing legalised abortion in Ireland. We are still hearing stories of women who suffered through Ireland's deeply cruel system of mother and baby homes and Magdalene laundries. More recently, we have heard from brave women like Vicky Phelan, who told their stories in relation to the Cervical Check service in Ireland.

These women had smear tests and were given results, saying no abnormalities were detected. Later audits of their results showed them to be incorrect. Still, this news was kept from the women for years, meaning that their cancer went undetected for many women, including Phelan. By the time they got a diagnosis, the disease was well advanced. Many of these women have since died. Vicky Phelan shone a bright and angry light on this scandal, highlighting that there is still a culture of paternalism to women's health care in Ireland for all our progress.

Stories matter. All stories matter. Yours matter as much as mine do. And we are the only ones who can articulate our stories with honesty and clarity. Our experiences are often radically different to men's. The narrative of "women's stuff", "women's problems" is damaging and has forced us together into a space we just share with each other.

Aside from the recent arrival of social media, the other place where women traditionally shared their stories was in fiction. And guess what? We get a genre all of our own. Once again, we are corralled together into something called "women's fiction", which is an improvement on the reductive "chick lit", but not by much. Apparently, this is important in case some man might accidentally pick up a book by a woman writer on his rush through an airport bookshop. Because men like to read literary works, which they think can only be written by other men. Women are writing about women's stuff... You know, domestic dramas and the like.

It has been remarked that if the book "Brooklyn" had been written by Colleen Toibin instead of Colm Toibin, it wouldn't even have been reviewed. Marian Keyes, one of Ireland's most beloved and successful writers, who has sold more than 33 million books, has also spoken about sexist attitudes to women writers and how women are assumed not to be able to write comedy. Although with brilliant writers such as Lisa McGee and Sharon Horgan writing some of the best TV comedy right now, that might be slowly changing (she types hopefully, although not entirely convincingly).

But the point is that stories have power. So, sisters, start speaking your truth publicly, loudly. Tell your story. Find your voice. Society tells women repeatedly that our power is based on how we look. That's a lie. Our power is in what we say. Our power is in our stories, which reflect our lived experiences. Most of our stories are not earth-shattering. Most of them are ordinary and mundane, but they matter. Other women need to hear them to know that what they have experienced or are experiencing isn't unique. Men need to hear them, too, so that our lived experience can become part of the national conversation. And that is where change begins.

# CONFIDENCE CRISIS

Are women generally less confident in their abilities than men, or is it just that we appear less confident because we are less comfortable with self-promotion? We need to look carefully at bringing up our girls and our boys. With our girls, we still tend to praise them for looking so pretty, and we encourage them to be gentle, considerate and generous, which is good but unbalanced. Boys tend to be praised for being strong and active and leaders. These attributes help them in the world men have created, which is also good but equally unbalanced.

Being combative in the boardroom does not come naturally to many women. And one has to ask, is it the right way to run a board meeting anyway? Successful women also often suffer from "imposter syndrome" in a way that many men don't. Women have also learned in the more recent past that working hard is no guarantee that you will succeed, so we still have fewer women in positions of power in companies and politics. From bitter experience, women generally think we have to be better than men to be equal to them.

I have often been in a TV or radio studio with my notes and my research to back up my argument, which

I have rehearsed in the car on the way in. Nine times out of 10, male panellists will wander in, just in the nick of time, exuding confidence and without a note in their hand. They wing it quite successfully. We over-prepare because we fear that we won't be treated as equal to men unless we are better than the men.

And, of course, we have to make sure we look as presentable as possible before putting ourselves out there for public dissection. I have repeatedly said that women are judged first on their looks and not on their achievements, so most women will have a professional blow dry and possibly professional make-up before a TV or public appearance. So, if your job includes performing as an MC, as a woman, you already have quite a time and financial commitment to make before ever taking to a stage!

Now, I know you can ask why we do this to ourselves, and I have to say that part of me wonders that too. However, having been on the receiving end of "comments"' (insults) about having the absolute gall to appear in public with our hair like that, or that fat, or that old, I tend to take all the help I can get. It's the old Ginger Rogers thing of having to do everything the guys do but backwards and in heels. I don't do heels, but you know what I mean.

Now, let me be clear, most women I know like to look their best. It does feel good to have your hair and make-up attended to professionally. Nevertheless, it bugs me that there doesn't seem to be a choice. For those who would prefer to do other things with their time and money, it is almost impossible to be your authentic self, especially when on TV. Mary Beard, who I quoted earlier, is a renowned historian and academic. She has suffered horrendous abuse when she has appeared on TV, mainly because she wears her hair longer than is deemed acceptable at her age, and, shock horror, she doesn't dye it or use make-up either. She is a woman at the height of her power and seems entirely comfortable in her own skin, but, apparently, she is fair game because she doesn't conform to how a woman of her age should look. This is deeply disturbing.

Equality is about choice. Women should be the ones to decide how we should present ourselves to the world, as should men. It should not be remarkable if a woman chooses not to have a full face of make-up on or her hair dyed or wear high heels. Of course, equally, it should be unremarkable if a woman looks fabulously coiffured because, ultimately, it's just not that important.

# FROM WICKED WITCHES TO IRISH MAMMIES

The woman was represented by the Triple Goddess of maiden, mother, and crone in ancient mythology. The maiden was revered for her physical youth and beauty. The mother was respected as the nurturer and carer. The crone was esteemed for her wisdom. With her decades of life experience, the crone was well versed in the ways of the world and the natural world in particular. She was a powerful woman in the community.

This wise and powerful woman was hijacked and recast as an evil spinster, capable of knowing the unknown and of dastardly deeds. In the Middle Ages, she became a witch with evil powers, but at least she had power.

Were witches the last truly visible expression of crone wisdom and power? Witches, who bore little resemblance to the cruel caricature we know today, were wise women in their communities who held a power that deeply unsettled the patriarchal establishment. But the word "witch" is regularly still used when describing an older woman, who perhaps lives life to her own tune. Someone who generally isn't bothered by what others think of her. Today we are more likely to hear such a person described as "a mad old witch."

Of course, the mad old witch most likely lives alone, well, except for the company of her cat or cats. And that right there is another older woman stereotype. The Crazy Cat Lady. This woman is most likely a "spinster". A woman who has never married and whose house is full of cats. The general implication of this description is that her personal and household hygiene is most likely a bit suspect. God help women who never marry – sure, only a cat or a clowder of cats could love her.

And of course, spinsters are always "the lonely old spinster". I mean, what woman would choose to live alone without a (presumably male) partner? Lots of women, it turns out. But spinsters are usually lonely, apparently.

Finally, the classic Irish older woman stereotype is The Irish Mammy. Originally, this was the brainchild of a funny and talented Irish writer, Colm O Regan. Much of what he wrote about it in his 'Book of The Irish Mammy' had more than a hint of truth. But since his humorous and affectionate dig at mammies, the Irish Mammy has morphed into a charming but daft and old-fashioned older woman who can't use a computer, has no understanding of text-speak and regularly gets it wrong. She also has huge issues figuring out the TV and is obsessed with the hot press (or, as we call it in Ireland, the airing cupboard) and ensuring you have a jumper when you go out. She is clearly a bit soft in the head. She's loveable and funny, but she ain't that clever.

Of course, the most recent stereotype is a Karen. This was originally a meme given to white middle-class women, who were often racist. But now, if you are a middle-aged or older woman who speaks up for herself and complains (legitimately) about something, you will be referred to as a Karen. And yep, I have been called Karen on several occasions.

These stereotypes of older women may be amusing. They may even hold a grain of truth, but make no mistake, they also inject not only into our own psyche but also the psyche of society the idea that older women are unattractive and generally a bit dim. So, just as we come to the point of our lives where we have a rich history and archive of stories and experiences, we discover that we are past it. We are lovely and can be patronised ("but in fairness, she looks good *for her age*"), but we are not really to be taken that seriously.

The truth is that older women (let's take that as being 50 plus) are (and this quote is from Forbes) "super consumers... they are the healthiest... wealthiest and most active generation in history."

Women control anywhere from 80% to 95% of household purchasing decisions. Older women generally have more disposable income than younger women. So, although it may not feel it, we have power, albeit a soft power. Advertisers seem very slow to cop onto this fact, however. I might assume that that is because marketing companies are stuffed with young people, but that would be ageist, right? Maybe it is because older women, in particular, have a low threshold for bullshit. And so much advertising, especially aimed at older women, is complete bullshit.

## ANTI-AGEING

There is one thing that advertisers do target at older women, and we all know what that is. I will have to try very hard not to type these words in caps because, in my head, I am screaming them. And that is anti-ageing products and procedures.

Anti-ageing is a big business. It was estimated to be worth in the region of $43 billion globally in 2019, and this is estimated to rise to around $55 billion by 2024. Instead of conferring on us the dubious gift of eternal youth, it's my opinion that anti-ageing just relieves us of our hard-earned cash and, more importantly, chisels away at our self-esteem. Many women over 50 have spoken of feeling they have become invisible. Ageing for women is seen as entirely negative, so we are told we must fight to remain young, to the point of cutting and pasting our faces. So, although we are no longer at risk of being drowned or burnt at the stake, our power has been stripped away by the continuous undermining of who we are, with the unrelenting barrage of messages about fighting ageing.

Imagine if, as women, we learned to love ourselves as we are. Imagine if we celebrated our age with each passing year. Imagine if we looked in the mirror and said, "Wow, you are still here! You are wise, funny, clever, kind and important," instead of looking at a new wrinkle and wondering whether we will get another week out of our hair colour. We would have more cash in our pockets, but, more importantly, we would have our rightful power. A power that comes with wisdom borne of experience.

We live in a very ageist society. Age is seen as a burden as opposed to a wonderful achievement. To age is to fail. I believe it is up to older women to change this narrative because it is the one that hurts us most. We are the demographic where sexism and ageism collide. This is no accident. Because once you reach the place where you no longer give a fuck about who thinks you are attractive, who approves of you, or who even likes you, you will step into your full power as a woman. Is it any wonder that the patriarchy wants to keep us distracted about how we look?

It can be troublesome when an older woman realises her own power and uses it. I give you Mary McAleese. I give you Jane Goodall. I give you Vandana Shiva. I give you Mary Robinson. These women have not only realised their power, but they also have powerful voices, which they use all the time.

Writer Mohadesa Najumi said, "The woman who does not require validation from anyone is the most feared on the planet." As we enter into our crone period, this is where our power comes from; from not giving a flying fuck what others think of us. But this power will not be effective in driving change unless we find our voices, unearth our stories, and learn to share them outside our comfort zones.

# CONCLUSION

*"She remembered who she was, and the game changed."*

**Lalah Deliah**

Menopause is finally coming out of the shadows and being talked about. This is good. This is important. But with so much focus on the difficulties and challenges that can accompany the "change of life", we are in danger of terrifying women in their thirties and forties about what lies ahead. There is also not enough attention given to the fact that menopause is transient; it is a phase of life. Unlike the Christmas puppy, it's not forever. Women need to see menopause as a beginning, a gateway, difficult and all as it might be for some. And not all women have a horrific menopause. We are all different, so we all experience menopause differently. Some women actually negotiate it with relative ease.

So, let's continue to talk about menopause and how women can be supported, but let's not forget that, after menopause, life can be sweeter and more potent than it might have been for decades.

## WE ARE THE DAUGHTERS OF WITCHES

As the feminist saying goes, "we are the grand-daughters of the witches they couldn't burn." These so-called witches were often women who didn't conform to the day's societal (patriarchal) gender norms. They were accused of all kinds of evil deeds and killed in the most gruesome manner. Today, calling a woman a witch is an insult exclusively reserved for women, especially older women. Hilary Clinton was called "the wicked witch of the left" when she ran for the Presidency in the US. Today's witch is an evil old woman, usually with a huge nose and a penchant for riding through the skies on a broomstick, cackling as she goes. In fact, witches are practitioners of ancient pagan religion, and the term can describe both women and men.

I went through a phase about 15 years ago when I realised that I was done with being Catholic, wondering if I was actually pagan. I began reading about Wicca and realised that it offered a great deal about how to live and honour the earth, something we seem to need now more than ever.

I am no expert on Wicca, but it is not a formalised religion with a hierarchy of power and a set of commandments or rules to be followed. I like that. I also like the basic ideology, which can be summed up by their guiding phrase, "that it harms none, do as you will." And harming none does not just refer to people but includes the planet and all its creatures. Wiccans live in harmony with nature and mark the turning of the wheel of the year. They live naturally close to Mother Nature. This honouring of the earth and her creatures appealed hugely to me, but so did the fact that Wicca is a far more feminine spirituality than the patriarchal nature of most other religions. The Divine Feminine is missing from most major religions, which means that, like our society, they are out of balance, and they leave women without a spiritual connection they can easily relate to.

However, although I am still languishing without any spiritual system and any regular spiritual practice, there is much I take from Wicca, including the idea that whatever energy you put out into the universe will return to you threefold. In other words, karma, which as my eldest daughter might say, "can be a bitch."

So, as you cruise into the witching hours of your own life, make your own rules, as long as you harm none. Abandon what no longer resonates with you. You have undoubtedly spent years either doing what you needed to advance your career or bringing up children or a mixture of both. This is your time. This is the time to collect everything you have gathered and examine it closely.

Some of what you have gathered is bullshit. This bullshit ranges from the messages you got when you were a little girl around being nice and gentle, to those you may have picked up at work, when your ideas were hijacked by male colleagues or when you were sabotaged by your own imposter syndrome; and from putting your needs last on your priority list to being available 24/7 to your children and or partner. Now it is time to dump what no longer serves you. Now is the time to dream again, but this time with added urgency as you become aware of a clock gently ticking in the wings of your life. This doesn't necessarily mean leaving home and heading off to live in Tibet, although if that floats your boat, I say go for it. However, what it does mean is listening to and reviewing your stories. Interrogate your dreams in a very real way. Work out what you want from this last big active phase of your life. It means beginning to find a way to make all that work. Become the woman you were always meant to be. And she may remind you very much of the girl you once were.

One of my feminist heroes, Gloria Steinem, said, "Remember when you were nine or 10, and you were this independent little girl climbing trees and saying, 'I know what I want, I know what I think'? That was before gender descended for most of us." She went on to say, "Ironically, I found by 60 you're free again. So, you're the same person you were at nine or 10, only now you have your own apartment, you can reach the light switch, you hopefully have a little money. So, you can do what you want."

# HEALTH REALLY IS WEALTH

If you really want to grab the opportunity in your fifties, sixties and seventies of making some of your dreams a reality, you must pay attention to your health. You wouldn't expect to drive a car for ten years without ever checking its oil and whatever else you have to check-in cars.

As my GP said, you can get away with an unhealthy lifestyle until you stop getting away with it. I went from normal blood sugar levels to diabetic levels in the space of 18 months. If, as you read this, you think that my previous lifestyle sounds a bit like yours, then I urge you to go to your GP and arrange a blood test. The problem with Diabetes is that you can have it for years with no major symptoms, and during that time, the high levels of sugar in your blood are possibly damaging your heart, your eyes, your kidneys, and other organs.

Losing weight and getting active is not about how you look. It is about staying healthy. You have stuff to do. You need to be healthy and fit to do it. Regular health check-ups should become a part of your life if they haven't already.

Type 2 Diabetes gave me the kick in the arse I needed to sort my shit out. Well, some of my shit. I am still a hot mess in various other areas of my life. But I am a changed woman. I am still a bit fat but not as fat, and I am much fitter. My body is happier. My new lifestyle and (modest) weight loss have generally made me feel younger, and if a happy fatty like me can make major changes and lose two stone in weight, then anyone can. The biggest obstacle to making the changes is often your own mind. Once I learned to control my brain, things became a lot easier. And again, that isn't as complicated as you might think. It is merely a case of telling your mind (yes, sometimes out loud) to shut up because you aren't listening to its enticements and temptations.

Being a powerful older woman is easier if you are fit and relatively healthy. Hopefully, it will make the "real" ageing (like when you are 80) a little easier.

# CARING

As our parents live longer than any previous generation, caring for a frail elderly parent or relative can be a huge issue that can come into your life just when you are beginning to taste the freedom of the post-menopausal years. Although there are men who are carers, the majority are women.

Caring is completely undervalued and something that really is invisible in our society. My years working for The Alzheimer Society of Ireland gave me a clear insight into the work involved in caring for someone. Many carers do what they do because they want to love their mother/father/spouse. What we need, of course, is far more support for those caring. Carers should at least be able to access regular respite breaks and have help daily from community care workers.

However, even though you might feel very stuck right now with this new burden, please don't sacrifice yourself completely if you can help it at all. Caring is often left to a daughter, and women can be bad at asking for help. Insist that your siblings row in to the care of a parent too.

It is important to clarify your priorities because I know that women caring for a frail parent can feel torn when their adult or near-adult children, or indeed their partner, need their support. Establish your priorities so that in your head, you won't feel pulled every way. It could, for instance, be kids first, followed by your partner and then the parent.

Women in their fifties and sixties or beyond can also find themselves caring for grandchildren, perhaps more than they would like. When I became pregnant at 25 and was on my own, my dear mother clearly said she would give me all the support she could, but she would not be doing full-time childcare regularly. At the time, I thought it was a bit harsh, but she was absolutely right. She had just started her own business and had things to do. I totally respect her for having the courage to be so honest.

No matter what kind of caring you might find yourself doing, please also make time for yourself. When you are on a flight, the safety demo will tell you that you must first attend to your own oxygen mask before helping others. You need to be healthy in mind and body to provide care for others. So, make time for your exercise, downtime, and social life.

## SILVER WOMEN

Nora Ephron, one of my favourite writers, once said

"There's a reason why 40, 50 and 60 don't look the way they used to and it's not because of feminism or better living through exercise. It's because of hair dye. In the 1950s only seven per cent of American women dyed their hair; today there are parts of Manhattan and Los Angeles where there are no grey-haired women at all."

All that money, time and chemical application we women spend on trying not to succumb to ageing; in attempting to hold onto our youth because grey hair is "so very ageing". But is it? Really?

Grey hair is a feminist issue, just like pockets. Up until recently, women's clothes came without pockets. I don't know what the thinking behind that was, but I can only presume men were given pockets because they didn't have handbags. But handbags aren't practical when rushing about in the office or at home. Women need pockets too.

Anyway, back to grey hair. As men age, they generally embrace their grey hair and become "silver foxes" – I give you George Clooney or Pierce Brosnan or Jon Bon Jovi. Men who dye their hair as they age generally get a hard time. I give you Mr Travolta (until he shaved it all off) or Mr Tom Jones until he copped on and embraced his grey. And then there's Mr Trump. The most uncool man on the planet with the daftest dyed barnet. Cool men don't dye. They can age without society commenting and urging them to fight ageing. They become silver foxes and elder statesmen. Women, however, are expected to rage against ageing and even when they do, they still apparently become invisible.

When I was a kid, I used to dream about being able to become invisible and what great craic that would be. I could listen in to all kinds of conversations that were verboten. I could go anywhere I wanted, sneaking onto trains and even planes. Best of all, I could get away with stuff because, as I mentioned earlier, I have always been highly visible because of my height. So, suffice to say that I have never felt invisible, even when I wanted to.

In more recent years, as I attempted to reinvent myself from a housewife and stay-at-home parent into a writer and broadcaster, I often found myself at events where I knew no one. Even though I am an extrovert and a bit of a show-off, I find those kind of situations difficult, precisely because I feel as if I am like a lighthouse shining a beacon over everyone else's head that says, "I know no one, and I wish I could just blend into the wall instead of feeling so very conspicuous."

As I enter my sixties, I still don't feel invisible. So I'm puzzled why many older women do feel this way.

Various studies have reported on this phenomenon, although they most often seem to be conducted on behalf of companies with skin (or hair) in this particular game, such as cosmetic companies or beauty clinics. Even some female celebrities have expressed the notion that after 50, they become invisible. I can understand this because, for women of a certain age, in the world of movies, meaty and leading roles for older women can be fairly thin on the ground. Indeed, closer to home, how many women over 60 do we see on our TV screens? Lots of older men but not as many older women. This is beginning to change, especially since women have taken TV stations to court for being sidelined once they reach a certain age. However, like most elements of our road to equality, the change is slow. Too slow. And this is possibly another reason why many older women feel invisible. We generally don't see ourselves reflected powerfully in our media – especially our broadcast media.

Some older women report feeling invisible when it comes to men. They do not command the attention of men in the way they did in their earlier decades. They go into a bar and wait longer to be served than they might have had to when they were younger women. I get that. Of course, I do.

Let me share something I learned shortly after turning 50, which was ten years ago. In the early days of my reinvention from housewife into a writer, I was invited onto a national late-night TV current affairs programme to do the newspaper review. Once I got over the shock of being asked and had verified that it was ME they were looking for and hadn't mixed me up with someone else, I tried to calm my nerves and got myself out to the TV studio. I had done my best to look presentable, but I was immediately taken into make-up, where my hair and face were attended to like all guests. I couldn't believe the transformation. I looked really fabulous in a way I hadn't for years. It didn't stop one nice man on Twitter (yes, I checked the show's hashtag afterwards) asking, "who was the fatty doing the paper review?" Oh, the judgement of any woman who dares put her head above the parapet, especially an older woman, and most especially a fat woman. Anyway, I digress. Again.

After that, I did more TV, mostly on a daily women's panel programme. I was often the oldest panellist. Each time, I dressed carefully and had the attention of the wonderful TV hair and make-up department, helping me to look my best. But I soon learned that my best is still quite short of my younger colleagues, who looked fabulous in a way I used to when I was in my twenties or thirties. I quickly decided not to physically compare myself with these younger women because they would always win. They had the younger, tighter skin and no middle-age flab. The years had yet to soften and line their faces. But I had decades of experience and tales to tell. They still had yet to collect some of theirs. In short, I had better stories. That was my worth to the programme. And in general, it's our greatest value as we age: our stories, experience, and wisdom.

You have read some of my stories. I haven't toured the world or gone on fantastical adventures. No, like most women's, my stories are the stuff of life. Each story, each experience is grafted into my personality. Some experiences may have made me angry, sad, or very happy, but all of them were important, just like yours. It doesn't matter if you were a rocket scientist, President of Ireland or a housewife. Your stories are part of the tapestry of the lived experience of being a woman. They are important. You should not be afraid to tell them.

I am not saying for a minute that you should abandon all care about how you look as you age. No. I am saying that the sooner you make peace with the fact that you are getting older, the better your experience of ageing will be. Our society is still largely patriarchal, even though much of what hobbles women is not as obvious as it was in the past. Now it's hidden just below the surface, a kind of unconscious sexism, and a big part of this is keeping women constantly distracted by how they look. Western society mainly still judges women by their appearance first, regardless of their achievements. Is it any wonder that so many older women feel invisible? We are told that we are invisible and that we have failed by showing our age.

Imagine for a moment if we turned the tables on this bullshit. Imagine if old age was lauded and commended. Imagine if it was youth that was seen as negative? Imagine if your daughters were being told to "fight youth" and sold all kinds of chemicals and even surgeries to achieve this? We, their mothers, would rightly be up in arms.

So why do we buy into the notion that to age is to fail, particularly for women? Why do we accept that our worth is primarily about how we look? Feminism is surely about equality for women. And equality means choice. If you want to have a few injections of Botox or dye your hair back to the colour it was in your twenties or thirties, you should go ahead. My problem is being told constantly that we aren't good enough as we are – being told to change how we look to be acceptable. As we age, this sexist nonsense is joined by the ageism that underpins the campaign to get women to "fight ageing". This is a pointless exercise for women, but one that keeps many companies making lots of money and keeps women from reaching their full power.

I don't want to live in the world described by Nora Ephron, where there are no silver-haired women. I want a world where I can see the grandmothers, the crones, the wise older women. I want a world where, at the very least, you are not told that your silver hair or laughter lines are "ageing" because they are not. It's the passage of time that is ageing. We are all ageing and have been since the day we were born. As we go beyond our childbearing years, we bear the physical marks of that ageing. We can choose to spend money and energy hiding our age with hair dye and Botox, but it doesn't change this fact.

I say to women of all ages, but particularly women over 50, don't be defined by your age, but equally don't deny it. Every year we get older is a triumph. Imagine what those who died young would have given to have silver hair, lines on their faces and age-spotted hands?

I have written most of this book as the world wrestled with COVID-19, which has been a sledgehammer in our lives, disrupting and destroying as it rampaged across the world. But there have been some upsides. Thanks to repeated lockdowns, my face is now framed in silver. I could say grey, but let's change that too. It's silver.

As you know, I experimented with "going lighter" a few years back, and I hated it. I didn't recognise myself when I looked in mirrors, so I had it dyed back to what used to be my natural colour: dark brown. I knew that there would come a day when I decided to stop when nature would prevail. I just hadn't thought it would come so soon, but thanks to COIVD-19, I now know how I look with silver hair. And I am surprised to realise that I like it.

Yes, I look my age, but so what. I have never lied about my age. I have no wish to be younger than I am. I wish for good health to allow me to make the absolute best of the next decade. We may have our most important work to do, not just for our daughters, but for our granddaughters in this next phase of life.

Again, Gloria Steinem said, "Women grow more radical with age. Someday an army of grey-haired women may quietly take over the earth." Thanks to a pandemic and the closure of hairdressers, I like to think that the day Steinem talked about may be on the horizon. Women are reclaiming their silver hair. My hope is that along with this, they will also reclaim their power. We owe it to our daughters and granddaughters to give the patriarchy one powerful kick without having to care as much about consequences.

My hair has become a metaphor for this new phase of life that I am almost ready to embrace. My silver hair changes me. However, unlike when I experimented with going slightly blonde, I recognised this new me. I know her. I have been waiting for her. Now that she is here, I find that I like her.

Silver has always been my choice for jewellery. Perhaps it's the old hippie in me, but I have always preferred it to gold. Silver is the colour of the moon and the ebb and flow of the tides. Colour psychology says it is soothing, calming, and purifying. It signals a time of reflection and change as it illuminates the way forward. I love that. Reflecting on a lifetime of changes. Rebirthing my true self. And illuminating the way forward for those who will follow us.

# THE WISDOM OF AN OLD OWL

Some years ago, himself gave me a gift of a Hawk Walk deep in the countryside in County Wicklow. It was a wonderful day spent learning about and being up close and personal with birds of prey and owls. When our session was over, our falconer led us out of the yard where all the birds were kept. On the way out, he stopped to introduce us to a huge owl sitting on a tree stump at the door to the cottage office.

He handed me a glove and carefully manoeuvred this large bird onto my arm while explaining that this was a "rescue owl" who had not been properly looked after – it had been fed processed meat and was thus a bit of a couch potato. She could fly – but generally didn't bother. Her hunting instincts were all gone through years of being "a pet".

The more the falconer explained about this bird, the more I realised I had met a kindred spirit. This was a mature, overweight owl who had forgotten her own magnificence and inherent wisdom through no fault of her own. I stroked her feathers, which were soft and downy. She turned to look at me, and we connected. Me and this owl, both of us with miles on the clock, with years of experience, and with all our sadness and our joy. We both wore all this on the outside. However, on the inside, we both knew that she was still a majestic bird, a hunter and thinker of deep thoughts. We gazed at each other, and our thoughts fused in the space between us.

"Yes," she said, "I am Owl. I can see the unseen. I can read the moon. I have stories. I am a wise old owl."

I often think of that wise old owl, sitting on her tree stump pondering all that life had taught her. In my mind, I see her fly at night, in the inky darkness, silently and invisibly into the woods where she communes with her owl sisters and brothers, sharing her wisdom, her stories and her experiences.

The Irish word for owl is *ulchabhán*, but colloquially owls were often called "cailleach oíche", which translates as "old women of the night", although cailleach is also the word for *witch*!

Best of all, a barn owl (or screech owl) is called a "scréachóg reilige", which is *screecher of the cemetery*. What better spirit animal for silver women reminding us to screech our truth at the cemetery of the patriarchy.

Turkish writer and thinker Murat ildan said, "The inauspiciousness of the owl is nothing but the inauspiciousness of the man who thinks that owl is inauspicious". And that is nothing compared to the inauspiciousness of men who think post-menopausal women are inauspicious, invisible, harmlessly batty or past our prime.

We are, in fact, busy remembering who we truly are and what it is that we really want, for ourselves, for our daughters and granddaughters and for the world. Like my owl friend, we are wising up to our true power and wisdom.

One day, we may indeed form an army to take over the world.

# ABOUT THE AUTHOR

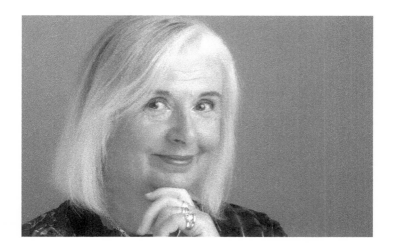

Barbara Scully is a writer, columnist and broadcaster. Her travel writing *and opinions* are frequently published in Ireland's national press and magazines. She is a regular on TV and radio, contributing to talk shows and with a regular weekly 'agony aunt' slot on the Moncrieff Show on Newstalk radio.

Barbara's 'portfolio career' was entirely accidental and included time in PR, travel and computer training.

Barbara is married to the photographer Paul Sherwood. They have three daughters, two grandchildren, a dog, four cats, and a resident fox in their garden near Dun Laoghaire, in County Dublin.

Printed in the USA
CPSIA information can be obtained
at www.ICGtesting.com
LVHW041300190923
758517LV00002BA/108